J. A. JACKSON

The Sweet Pepper Cajun! Tasty Soulful Food Cookbook!

Southern Family Recipes!

Copyright © 2019 by J. A. Jackson

All rights reserved. No part of this publication may be reproduced, stored or transmitted in any form or by any means, electronic, mechanical, photocopying, recording, scanning, or otherwise without written permission from the publisher. It is illegal to copy this book, post it to a website, or distribute it by any other means without permission.

This novel is entirely a work of fiction. The names, characters and incidents portrayed in it are the work of the author's imagination. Any resemblance to actual persons, living or dead, events or localities is entirely coincidental.

J. A. Jackson asserts the moral right to be identified as the author of this work.

J. A. Jackson has no responsibility for the persistence or accuracy of URLs for external or third-party Internet Websites referred to in this publication and does not guarantee that any content on such Websites is, or will remain, accurate or appropriate.

Designations used by companies to distinguish their products are often claimed as trademarks. All brand names and product names used in this book and on its cover are trade names, service marks, trademarks and registered trademarks of their respective owners. The publishers and the book are not associated with any product or vendor mentioned in this book. None of the companies referenced within the book have endorsed the book.

Photo Credits – All photos used Purchased From Deposit Photos com- https://depositphotos.com/

First edition

This book was professionally typeset on Reedsy. Find out more at reedsy.com

Dedicated to those who love soulful tasty foods from the heart!

Recipes were provided by Dorothy Henson, Lady D., Lady J, Lady V, Lady R , Jerreece Jackson and J. A. Jackson.

Come join us, grab a seat, fill a bowl, and take a taste of our scrumptious food. We believe food is our common ground and in flavor do we trust!

Lady J

Contents

Foreword	v
Preface	vi
Acknowledgement	vii
Breakfast/Brunch	1
Start Your Day Right! Breakfast!	3
Homemade Pancakes!	5
Perfectly Golden French Toast	8
Cajun Fluffy Scrumptious Scramble Eggs!	10
Cajun Spinach Quiche!	12
Cajun Sausage Potatoes Egg Bake!	14
Cajun Shrimp & Grits!	16
Basic Grits!	18
Cajun Breakfast Potatoes, w/Onions & Bell Peppers!	21
Cajun Fried Green Tomatoes!	23
Toss Green Salad	26
Cucumber & Onion Salad	28
Southern Yellow Mustard Potato Salad!	30
Louisiana Corn & Crab Bisque!	32
Cajun Lima Bean & Okra Soup!	34
Creole Soup!	35
Creole Roasted Garlic Soup!	37
Creole Simple Tomatoes Soup!	39
Old Fashion Green Beans!	41
Cajun Brussels Sprouts!	43
Cajun Spaghetti Supreme!	45
Cajun Garlic Spaghetti!	47

Cajun 4 Cheese Spaghetti!	49
Authentic Cajun Homemade Macaroni & Cheese!	51
Cajun Chicken Breast!	53
Cajun Fried Chicken!	55
Cajun Pan Seared Salmon!	57
Cajun Shrimp Sandwich!	59
Spicy Cajun Shrimp Sandwich W/Chipotle Avocado...	61
Cajun Catfish Tacos Deep Fried or Oven Baked	63
Fried Cajun Catfish!	66
Cajun Buttery Steak Bites!	71
Cajun Style Beef Tips & Rice!	73
Cajun Bone-In Rib Eye Steaks	75
Create Your own Rub: Cajun Seasoning!	78
Cajun Pork Chops!	82
Cajun Style Roast Pork!	84
Sweet Desserts!	86
Soft Sweet Molasses Cookies!	88
Southern Tea Cookies Recipe!	91
Homemade Moon Pies!	93
Moon Pie with a Chocolate Cookie!	97
Quick Semi Homemade Pie Crust Peach Cobbler!	99
Quick Apple Pockets!	101
Old Fashion Homemade Pecan Squares!	103
Semi Home-Made Quick Pecan Squares!	105
Homemade Old-Fashioned Lost Pies of the South!	107
Arkansas Black Apple Pie!	109
Old Time Pie Crust Made With Vinegar!	111
Lost Stacked Sweet Potato Pie Recipe!	113
Slap Ya Mamma Cajun Meat Pies!	116
Beverages/Drinks/Punches/Smoothies!	120
Tasty Watermelon Punch!	122
Fruity Homemade Punch!	124
Mock Champagne Punch!	127

Fruity Berry Smoothie!	131
Homemade Iced Tea!	134
Holidays & Special Occasions!	136
Southern Cornbread Dressing!	138
Sweet Candied Potatoes!	141
Creole Roast Turkey!	143
Hickory Smoked Bacon Collard Greens!	145
Angel Biscuits!	147
Pineapple Brown Sugar Glazed Ham!	149
Creamy Cheesy Scalloped Potatoes!	152
Roasted Holiday Veggies!	154
Butternut Squash & Andouille Dressing!	155
Cranberry Salad Mold!	157
Cranberry Pineapple Melody!	159
Mamma's Million Dollar Pound Cake!	160
30 Minutes Dinner Rolls!	164
Holidays Time For Family & Friends!	166
Traditional Southern New Year's New Dinner!	168
Traditional New Year's Pork Roast!	170
New Year's Good Luck Long Noodle Creamy Cajun Pasta!	173
Smoky Black-Eyed Peas!	175
Baked Silver Fish!	178
Smoky Collard Greens with Ham!	181
Golden Brown Cornbread!	183
New Year's Good Luck Almond Pound Cake!	185
Holiday Appetizer Party!	188
Cajun Mini Crab Cakes!	189
Cajun Stuff Mushrooms!	191
Cajun Oysters Spinach & Cheese!	193
Cajun Ham and Corn Beignets!	195
Cajun Crawfish Boulettes!	197
Cajun Spicy Appetizer Meatballs	200
Crispy Oven Friend Cajun Chicken Wings!	202

Cajun Pan Roasted Pumpkin Seeds!	204
Keep Calm and Cook On!	206
Come Join Us! Taste Our Scrumptious Food!	207
Young or Old Learning To Cook Can Be Fun!	209
Books by J. A. Jackson	210
About the Author	211
Also by J. A. Jackson	212

Foreword

Recipes were provided by Dorothy Henson, also known as Lady D, Lady V, also known as Viola Henson-Hazelwood. (my grandmother), Lady R also known as Ruby Jimmerson my other grandmother, Jerreece Jackson and J. A. Jackson.

Thank you to my mother Dorothy Henson, who wrote down many of the recipes you find here. I am so glad I encased those hand-written recipes into a notebook and saved them. They are the flavors; I cherish most from enjoying my mother's wonderful cooking. My mother as has my grandmothers have all been called home, but they left me with a wonderful legacy I share with you today.

Sorry to say there is no gentleman known as the Sweet Pepper Cajun, living, any longer but he left us all with his great wit and love of Southern cooking. Thank you, Daddy, Jerry O' for being my Sweet Pepper Cajun man.

Copyright law does not protect recipes that are mere listings of ingredients. These fine ladies shared their recipes with me as has many others in families large or small who pass recipes down, through generation after generation. With each new generation some changes are done to the old recipe to make it the new. With our family's discover of Slap Yo Mamma seasoning we have been adding it to most of our recipes because we love the taste, we know that taste as with most things are on an individual bases and one should always feel the need to use what one feels is there best seasoning ingredient. Therefore if you are not partial to Slap Yo Mamma Cajun seasoning, please feel free to use the seasoning of your choice.

Preface

Recipes were provided by Dorothy Henson, Lady D., Lady J, Lady V, Lady R , Jerreece Jackson and J. A. Jackson.

Photo Credits - All photos used Purchased From Deposit Photos com- https://depositphotos.com/ and from © Can Stock Photo

Acknowledgement

Recipes were provided by Dorothy Henson, Lady D., Lady J, Lady V, Lady R,
Jerreece Jackson aka J. A. Jackson.

This is dedicated to the cooks who came before me. That secret society of grandmothers, mothers, aunts, neighbors and church ladies. You know the ones who loved to cook, who had all their recipes etched into their memories, those ladies who could whip up a cake batter with just a folk. Who felt no shame in sharing their recipes and stories from the heart? These wonderful beings taught me to love what they cooked and to learn how to cook it for myself. Thank you to those fabulous ladies who shared their love for cooking great flavorful food with me and who taught me how to share, I now share their recipes with you. Enjoy.

Breakfast/Brunch

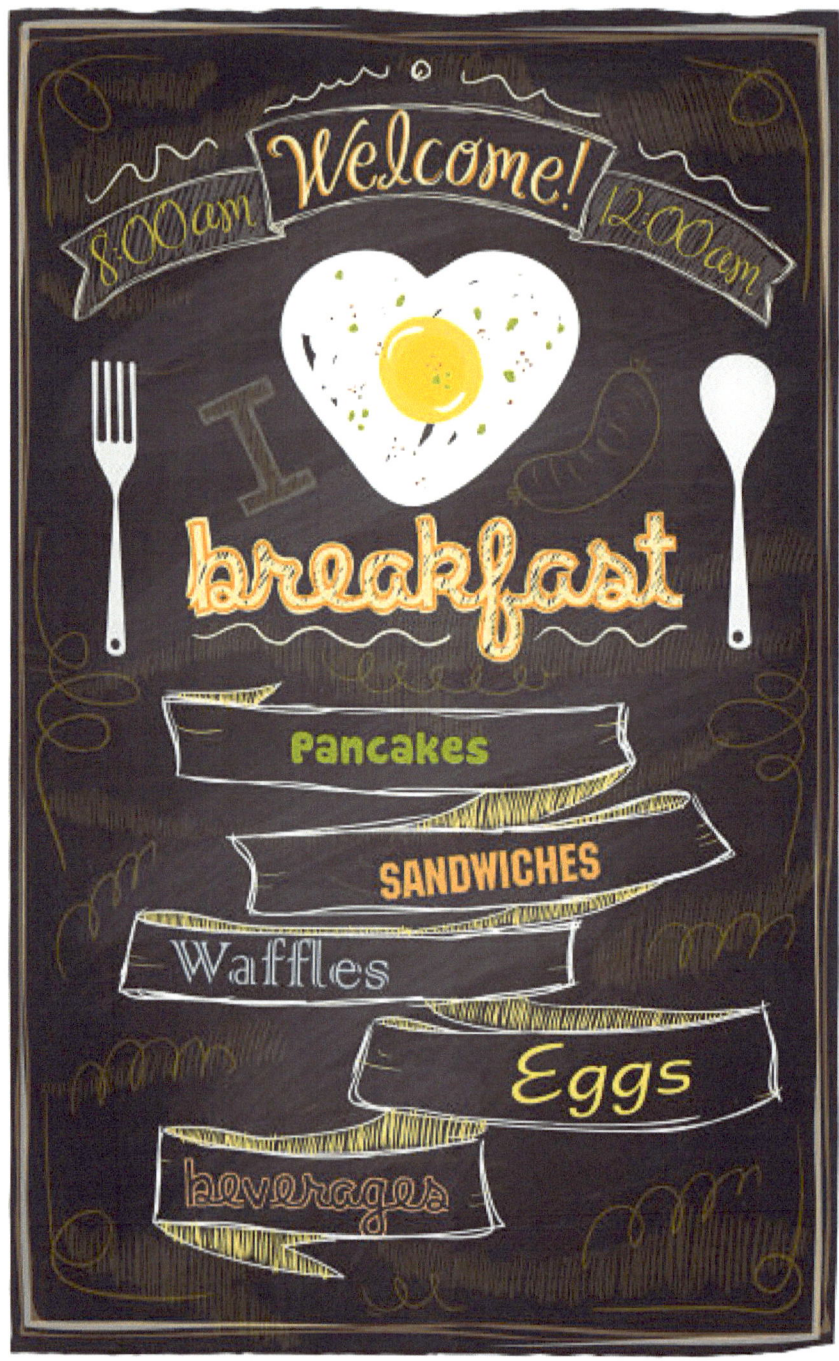

Start Your Day Right! Breakfast!

Add a Cajun Twist! These Biscuits are great for Breakfast and Brunch!

Homemade Buttermilk Biscuits

Preheat oven to 450°.

Ingredients:

- 2 cups all-purpose flour
  - 2 teaspoons baking powder
  - 1/2 teaspoon baking soda
  - 1/2 teaspoon salt
  - 1/4 cup shortening
  - 3/4 cup buttermilk

Directions:

*Turn oven down to 350 degrees.

In a bowl, combine flour, baking powder, baking soda and salt; cut in shortening until the mixture resembles coarse crumbs.

Stir in buttermilk; knead dough gently. Roll out to 1/2-in. thickness. Cut with a 2-1/2-in. biscuit cutter and place on a lightly greased baking sheet.

Bake until golden brown, 10-15 minutes.

Yes You Can Freeze Biscuits

***Freeze option**: Freeze cooled biscuits in a resealable freezer container. To use, heat in a preheated 350° oven 15-20 minutes.

* * *

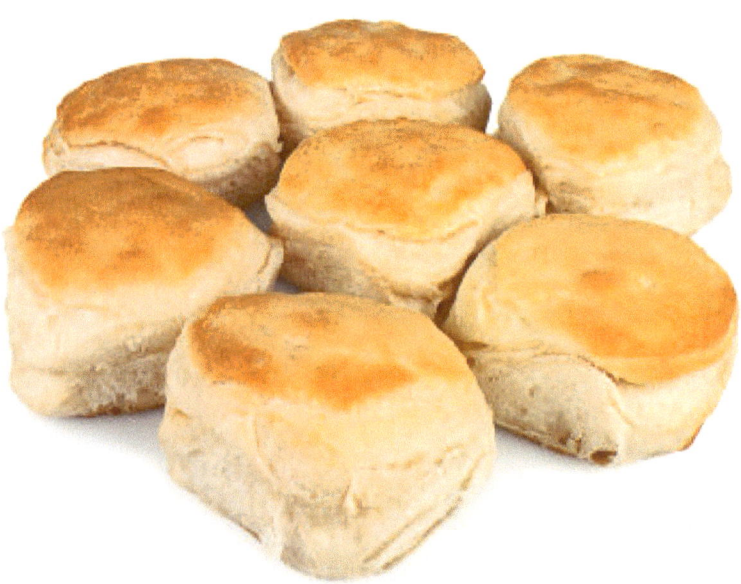

Always a morning favorite! Homemade Biscuits!

Homemade Pancakes!

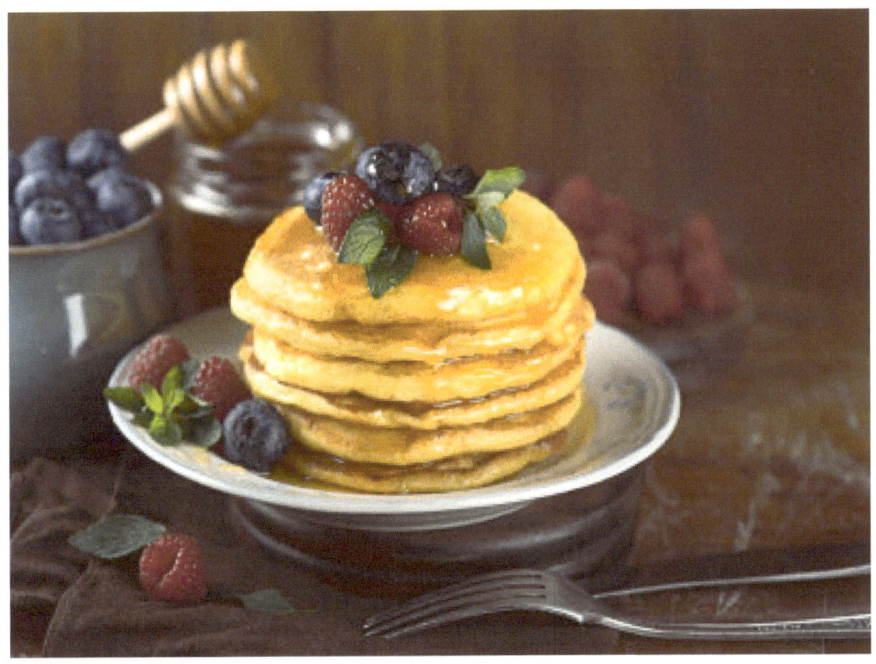

Delicious Home-made Pancakes

Homemade Pancakes

Ingredients:

4 cups all-purpose flour
- 1/4 cup sugar
- 2 teaspoons baking soda
- 2 teaspoons salt
- 1-1/2 teaspoons baking powder
- 4 large eggs, room temperature
- 4 cups buttermilk

Directions:

·In a large bowl, combine the flour, sugar, baking soda, salt and baking powder. In another bowl, whisk the eggs and buttermilk until blended; stir into dry Ingredients just until moistened.

·Measure out ¼ pancake mixture onto a lightly greased hot griddle; turn when bubbles form on top. Cook until second side is golden brown.

Flavor options...

· For Bananas flavored pancakes add one large mashed banana to wet mixture and stir of well blended.

·¼ Cup Chopped walnuts or pecans can be added to taste. (Either in wet mixture before cooking or as a topping after pancakes are done.)

·For cinnamon flavored pancakes add 1 teaspoon of cinnamon to taste. (Either in wet mixture before cooking or as a topping after pancakes are done.)

·For pumpkin flavored pancakes add ½ cup of mashed pumpkin and 2 teaspoons of ground cinnamon. (Add into wet mixture before cooking.)

Topping Options...

You can make these pancakes taste scrumptiously delicious and be uniquely yours when you add your favorite topping. Decorations suggestions: Top with your favored fresh berry. Strawberry, Raspberry, Blackberry or Blueberry will all add that special flavor taste kick, that your family and friends will love. If bananas and nuts are more your taste. Top with freshly sliced bananas or warm toasted pecans. Fresh warm sliced apple spice is always a treat.

Perfectly Golden French Toast

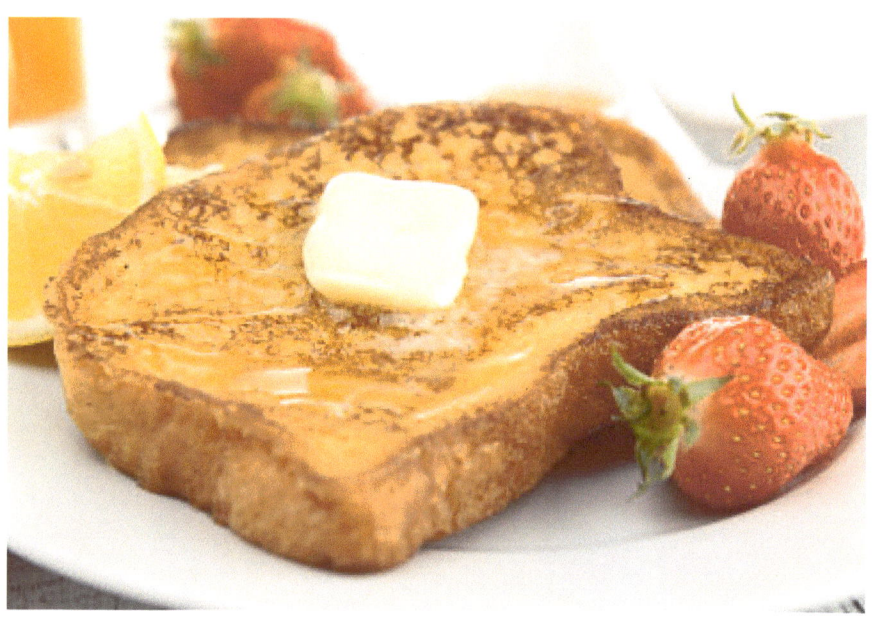

Tip: For the Best French Toast dip bread in mixture don't soak!

Perfectly Golden French Toast

Ingredients:

- 1/3 cup fresh orange juice
  - 1 teaspoon grated orange zest
  - 4 large eggs
  - 1/2 teaspoon ground cardamom
  - 1/4 cup butter, cubed
  - 12 slices day-old French bread (3/4 inch thick)
  - Maple syrup '

Directions:

- In a bowl, combine orange juice, zest, eggs and cardamom; beat well. Melt the butter in a 13 x 9-in. pan in the oven. Remove pan from oven. Dip the bread on both sides in the egg mixture; place in a single layer in pan. Bake at 450° for 10 minutes, turning once. Serve with syrup.

Cajun Fluffy Scrumptious Scramble Eggs!

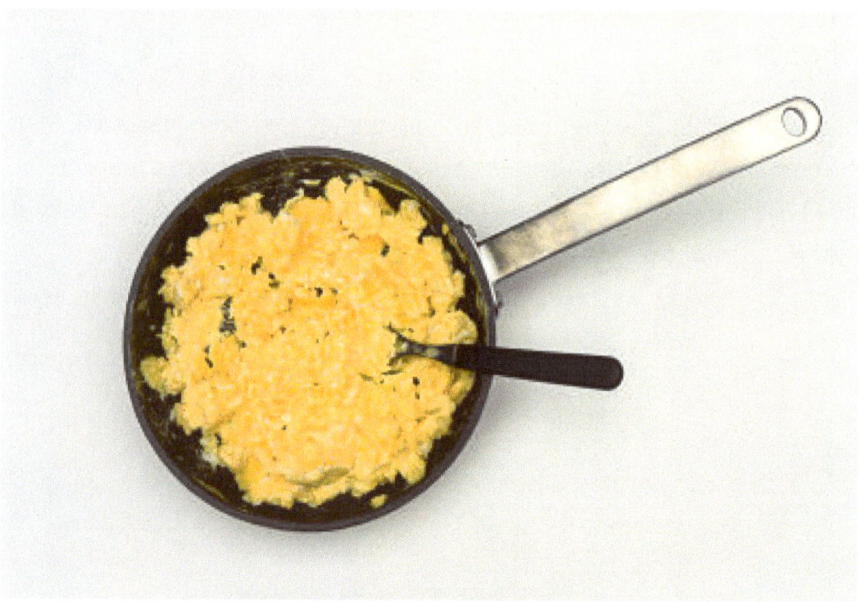

Fluffy Scrumptious Scramble Eggs!

Cajun Fluffy Scrumptious Scramble Eggs are great for breakfast or brunch!

Ingredients:

- 6 large eggs
  - 1/4 cup evaporated milk or half-and-half cream
  - 1/4 teaspoon Slap Ya Mama Cajun Seasoning (season to taste)
  - 1/8 teaspoon pepper
  - 1 tablespoon canola oil
  - 2 tablespoons process cheese sauce (optional)
  - 2 tablespoons chopped chives (optional for garnish)

Directions:

In a bowl, whisk eggs, milk, salt and pepper. In a large skillet, heat oil over medium heat. Pour in egg mixture; stir in cheese sauce. Cook and stir until eggs are thickened and no liquid egg remains.

Cajun Spinach Quiche!

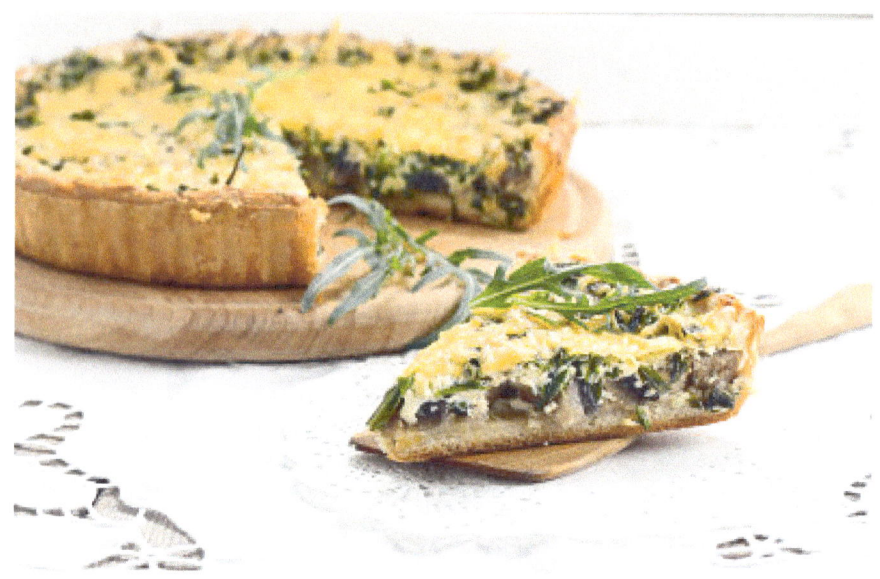

Brunch isn't complete without Cajun Spinach Quiche!

Ingredients:

- 1 cup chopped onion
  - 1 cup sliced fresh mushrooms
  - 1 tablespoon vegetable oil

CAJUN SPINACH QUICHE!

- 1 package (10 ounces) frozen chopped spinach, thawed and well drained
- 2/3 cup finely chopped fully cooked ham
- 5 large eggs
- 3 cups shredded Muenster or Monterey Jack cheese
- 1/8 teaspoon pepper (
- ¼ teaspoon Slap Ya Mama Cajun Seasoning (season to taste)
- Pinch of cayenne pepper (optional)

*Use 1 9 inch already prepared pie crust be sure to do Blind baking of pie crust * **Blind bake pie crust first before filing.**

Directions:

- In a large skillet, sauté onion and mushrooms in oil until tender. Add spinach and ham; cook and stir until the excess moisture is evaporated. Cool slightly. Beat eggs; add cheese and mix well. Stir in spinach mixture and pepper; blend well. Spread evenly into a per made pie crust or quiche dish. Bake at 350° for 40-45 minutes or until a knife inserted in center comes out clean.

***Blind baking pie crust.**

When a pie or tart filling is very wet, the crust must be prebaked before it is filled. This technique is called "blind baking," and it prevents the crust from becoming soggy. Quiche is one example of a tart that requires a prebaked shell because the custard filling is liquid in its raw state.

Cajun Sausage Potatoes Egg Bake!

Preheat oven to 350°.

Ingredients

- 1-pound lean ground sausage (can slice/dice sausage links or can substitute ground beef as a healthier choice)
  - 2 teaspoons onion powder
  - 1/2 teaspoon Slap Ya Mama Cajun Seasoning (season to taste)
- Pinch of cayenne pepper optional
- 1/2 teaspoons salt, divided
- 1 teaspoon garlic powder
- 1/2 teaspoon rubbed sage
- 1/2 teaspoon crushed red pepper flakes
- 1 package (10 ounces) frozen chopped spinach, thawed and squeezed dry
- 4 cups frozen shredded hash brown potatoes
- 14 large eggs
- 1 cup fat-free ricotta cheese
- 1/3 cup fat-free milk
- 3/4 to 1 teaspoon pepper
- 3/4 cup shredded Colby-Monterey Jack cheese
- 1-1/3 cups grape tomatoes, halved

Directions:

Preheat oven to 350°. In a large skillet, cook beef with onion powder, 1/2 teaspoon salt, garlic powder, sage and pepper flakes over medium heat 6-8 minutes or until no longer pink, breaking up beef into crumbles; drain. Stir in spinach. Remove from heat.

Spread potatoes in a greased 13 x 9-in. baking dish; top with beef mixture. In a large bowl, whisk eggs, ricotta cheese, milk, pepper and remaining salt; pour over top. Sprinkle with cheese. Top with tomatoes.

Bake, uncovered, 45-50 minutes or until a knife inserted in the center comes out clean. Let stand 5-10 minutes before serving.

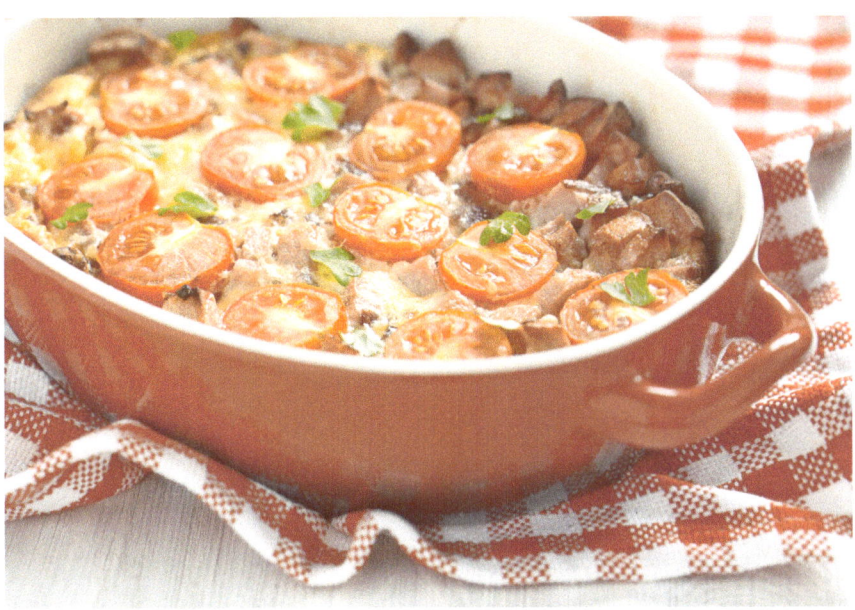

Make it your own - dice or slice your favorite breakfast meat to add to this dish!

Cajun Shrimp & Grits!

Ingredients:

- 2 cups reduced-sodium chicken broth
- 2 cups 2% milk
- 1/3 cup butter, cubed
- 3/4 teaspoon salt
- 1/2 teaspoon pepper
- 3/4 cup uncooked old-fashioned grits
- 1 cup shredded cheddar cheese
- **SHRIMP:**
- 8 thick-sliced bacon strips, chopped
- 1-pound cleaned peeled shrimp
- 3 garlic cloves, minced
- 1 teaspoon Slap Ya Mamma Cajun seasoning (season to taste)
- *pinch of cayenne pepper to taste * optional
- 4 green onions, chopped *optional garnish on top
- Make sure you clean shrimp before cooking or purchase already peeled shrimp at Wal-Mart Super Store approximately $10.00 per bag already cleaned & peeled large shrimp.
- 1 to 2 strips of fried bacon for garnish optional

Directions:

·In a large saucepan, bring the broth, milk, butter, salt and pepper to a boil. Slowly stir in grits. Reduce heat. Cover and cook for 12-14 minutes or until thickened, stirring occasionally. Stir in cheese until melted. Set aside and keep warm.

·In a large skillet, cook bacon over medium heat until crisp. Remove to paper towels with a slotted spoon; drain, reserving 4 teaspoons drippings. Sauté the shrimp, garlic and seasoning in drippings until shrimp turn pink. Serve with grits and sprinkle with onions.

** See how to cook Basic Grits recipes in Chapter 8**

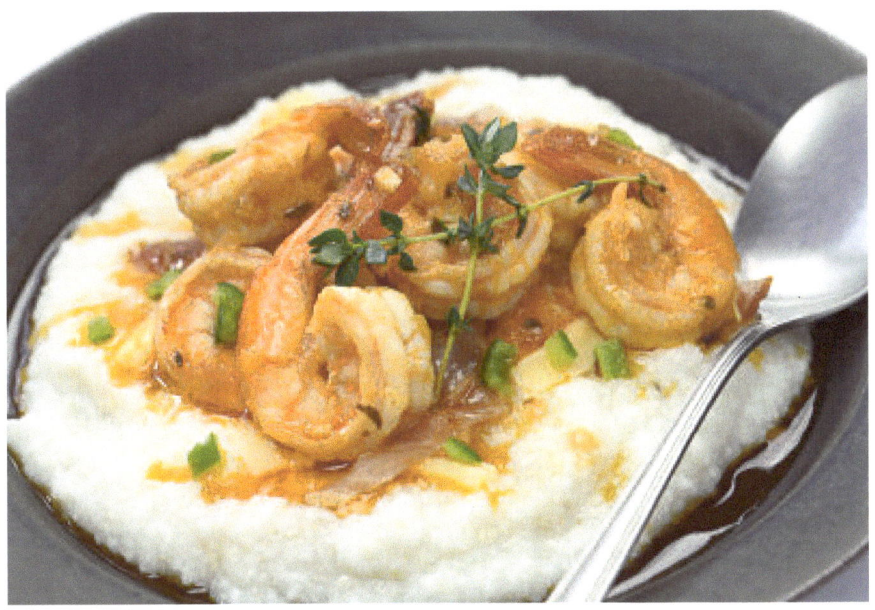

Southern Down Home Classic Shrimp & Grits!

Basic Grits!

Ingredients:

1 cup coarsely-ground grits 5 cups water or stock (4 1/2 if you want thicker grits) 1 teaspoon salt 4 tablespoons butter (or to taste, go with your heart)
for smaller portions see box of grits for measuring amounts

Directions:

·In a large, heavy-bottomed saucepan, bring the water to a boil. Bring the heat down to medium, so that the water simmers, then slowly whisk in the grits, stirring constantly until they begin to thicken (3-5 minutes).

·Reduce the heat to low, so that the grits bubble once or twice every few seconds but aren't rolling. Cook for 40-50 minutes (the coarser your grits are, the longer they need to cook), stirring frequently to make sure the grits aren't scorching on the bottom of the pan.

·Once the grits are tender and cooked through, beat in the butter and salt and serve hot.

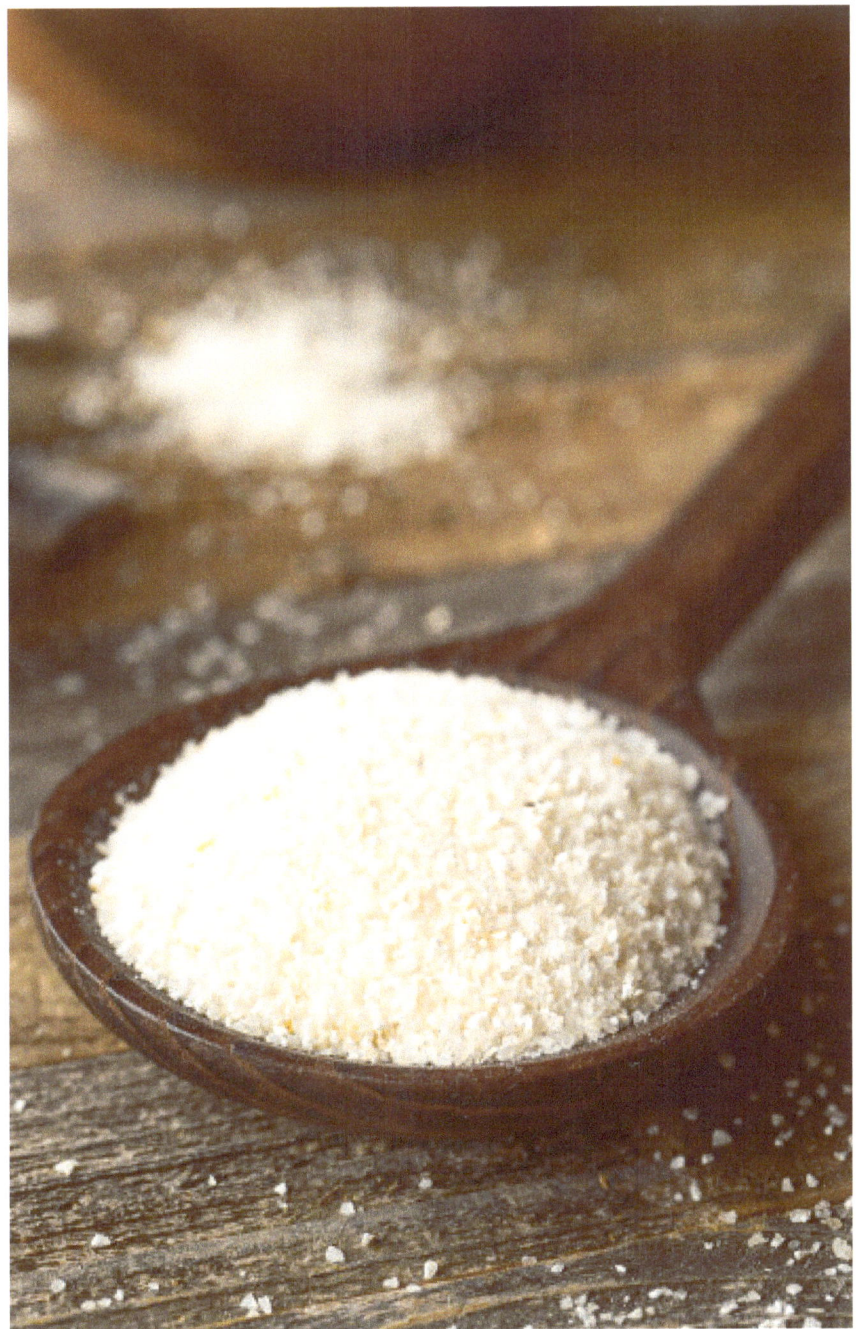

Grits is a food made from boiled cornmeal it is known to be a laid-back Southern comfort food!

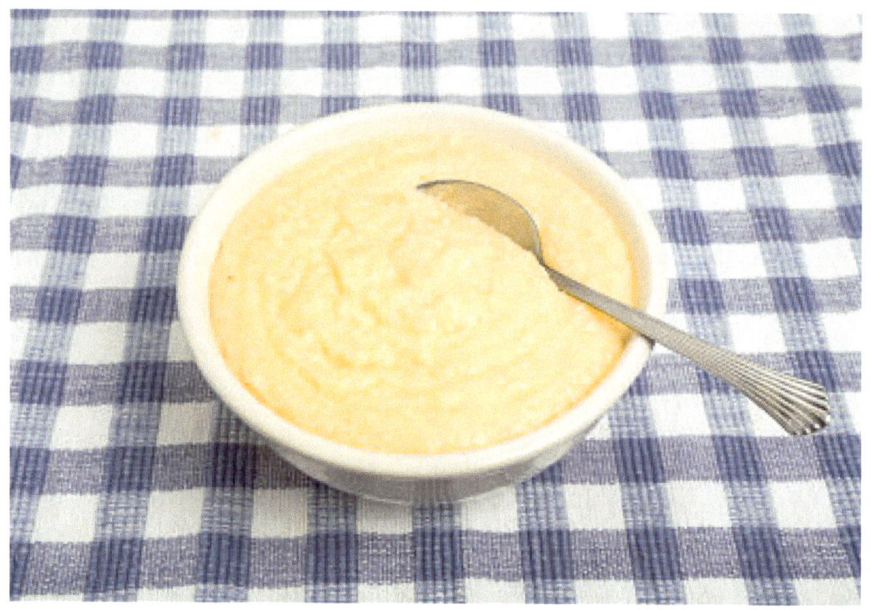

Basic bowl of grits can be topped with many foods... Cheese, Shrimp, Bacon, etc...

Cajun Breakfast Potatoes, w/Onions & Bell Peppers!

Ingredients:

2 Tbsp. olive oil
1 Tbsp. unsalted butter
4 large or 6 medium potatoes, peeled and cut into ½" cubes
1 onion, diced
1 red bell pepper, diced
2 tsp. fresh parsley, chopped
3 garlic cloves, minced
½ teaspoon Slap Ya Mamma Cajun seasoning (season to taste)
Pepper, to taste (*optional pinch of cayenne pepper)
1/4 cup chicken broth

Directions:

Preheat the oil and butter in a large nonstick skillet over medium heat. Add potatoes, toss to coat with oil, and place a lid on the pan. Allow the potatoes to cook covered for 10 minutes.

Remove the lid and increase the heat to medium high. Add onion and bell pepper. Cook for 15 minutes, stirring occasionally, until the potatoes and vegetables turn golden brown.

Add ½ teaspoon of Slap Ya Mamma Cajun Seasoning, the parsley and garlic and ¼ cup of chicken broth; cook for 2 minutes covered with lid to make sure potatoes are tender. Season with fresh cracked black pepper. *Optional –Sprinkle with Parmesan and serve immediately.

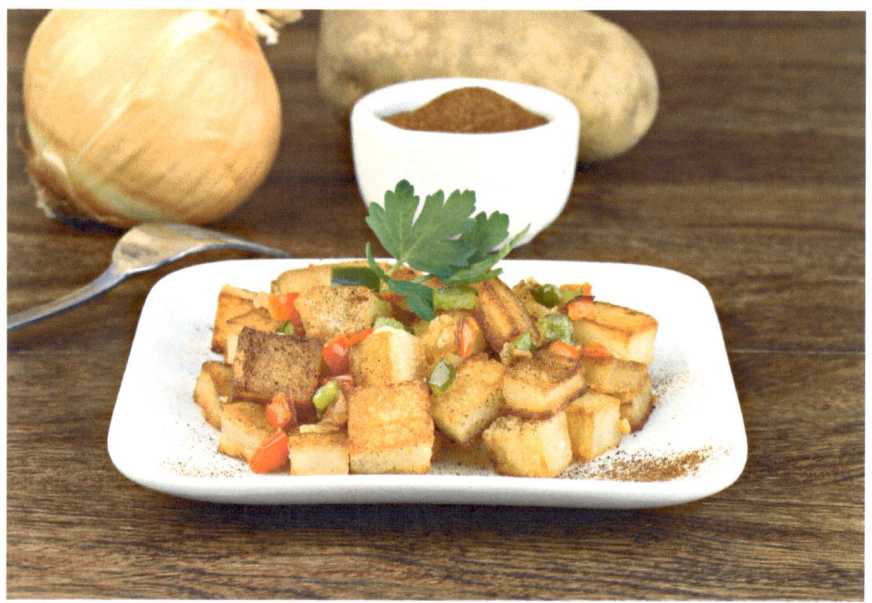

Cajun Fried Green Tomatoes!

Ingredients:

- 3/4 cup self-rising flour
- 1/4 cup cornmeal
- 1/2 teaspoon sugar
- 1 teaspoon Slap Ya Mamma Cajun seasoning (season to taste)
- 3/4 teaspoon cayenne pepper *optional* can substitute black pepper
- 1 egg
- 3/4 cup milk (add milk gradually as may not need to use as much)
- 4 medium green tomatoes, cut into 1/2-inch slices
- 1/4 cup canola oil to start

Directions:

- In a shallow bowl, combine the flour, cornmeal, sugar, salt and cayenne, and milk. Be sure to gradually add milk, as batter should resemble pancake batter. Pat green tomato slices dry. Working in batches, dip tomatoes slices in batter allow excess batter to drip back into the bowl.
- In a large nonstick skillet, heat 4 teaspoons oil over medium heat. Fry tomato slices, four at a time, for 3-4 minutes on each side or until golden brown, adding more oil as needed. Drain on paper towels.

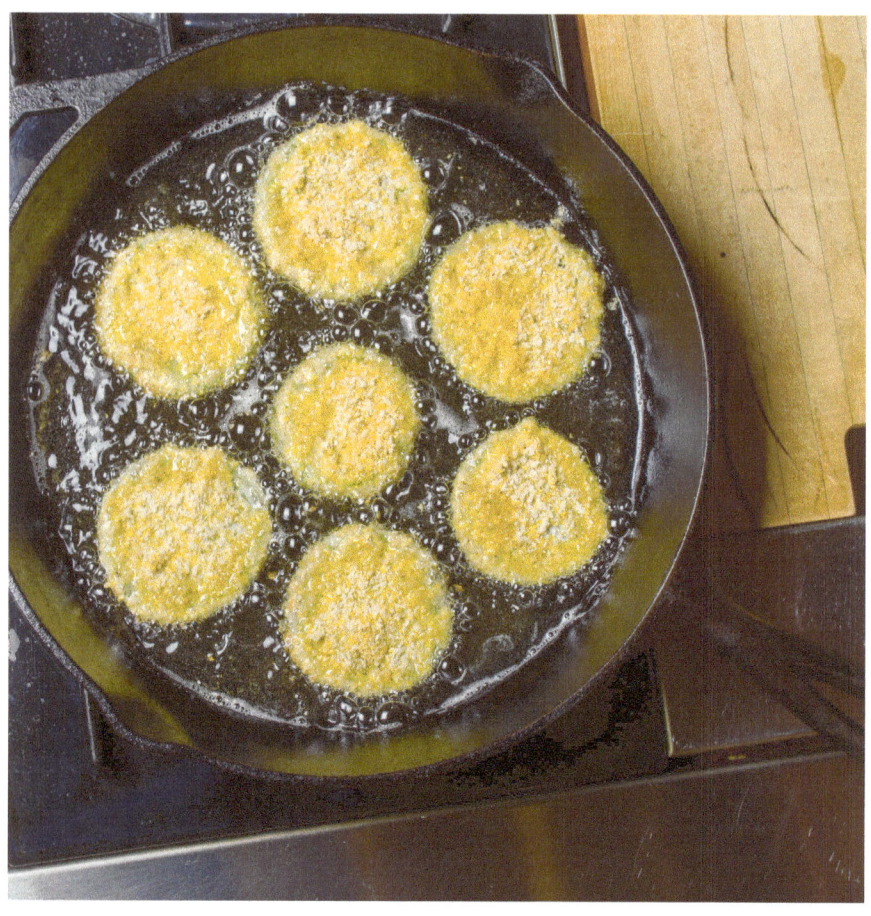

Fry with 1/4 cup canola oil, add more as needed.

CAJUN FRIED GREEN TOMATOES!

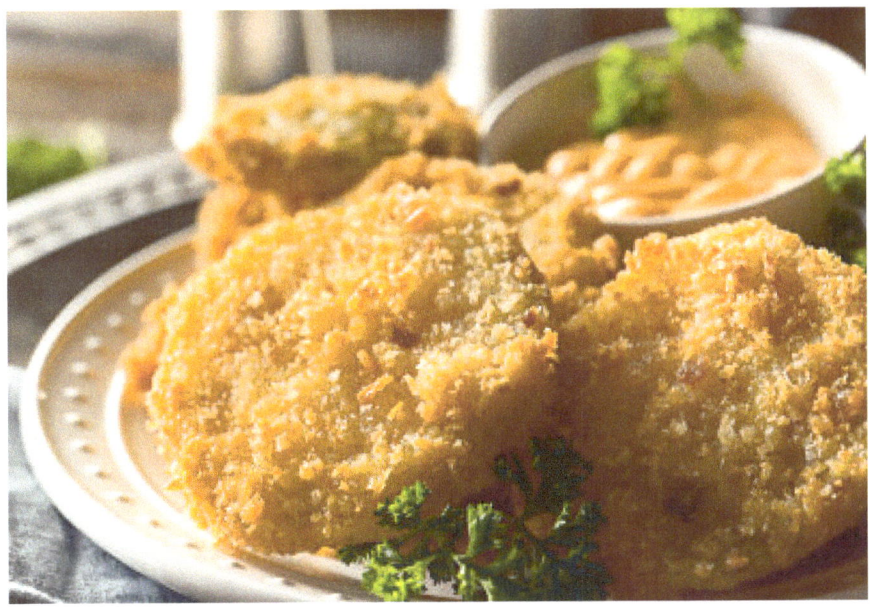

Fried Green Tomatoes served with my favorite dipping sauce, Thousand Island Dressing!

Toss Green Salad

Ingredients:

- 5 cups torn mixed greens
  - 1 medium tomato, diced (*or cherry tomatoes cut in half)
  - 1 cup sliced radishes
  - 1 cup sliced red onion
  - 1/4 cup bacon bits
  - 2/3 cup canola oil
  - 1/3 cup cider vinegar
  - 1-1/4 teaspoons Slap Ya Mamma Cajun seasoning (season to taste)
  - 1/2 teaspoon pepper

Directions:

- In a salad bowl, toss the first five Ingredients. In a small bowl, whisk the remaining Ingredients. Pour over salad and toss to coat.

TOSS GREEN SALAD

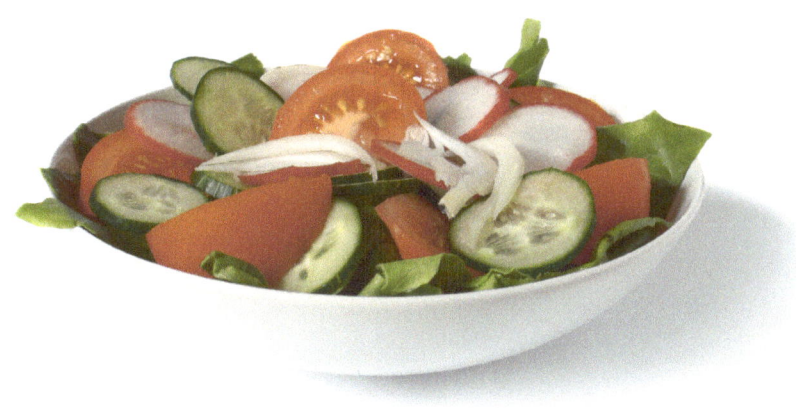

Cider Vinegar dressing optional, you can use your favorite salad dressing for this salad.

Cucumber & Onion Salad

Ingredients:

- 2 small English cucumbers, thinly sliced
  - 1 cup thinly sliced red onion
  - 2 tablespoons white wine vinegar or rice vinegar
  - 1 tablespoon white vinegar
  - 1/4 teaspoon Slap Ya Mamma Cajun seasoning (season to taste)
  - 1/4 teaspoon pepper
  - 1/4 teaspoon sesame oil

Directions:

- Place all Ingredients in a bowl; toss to combine. Refrigerate, covered, about 1 hour. Serve with a slotted spoon.
    note you can add fresh cut tomatoes to this recipe also.

CUCUMBER & ONION SALAD

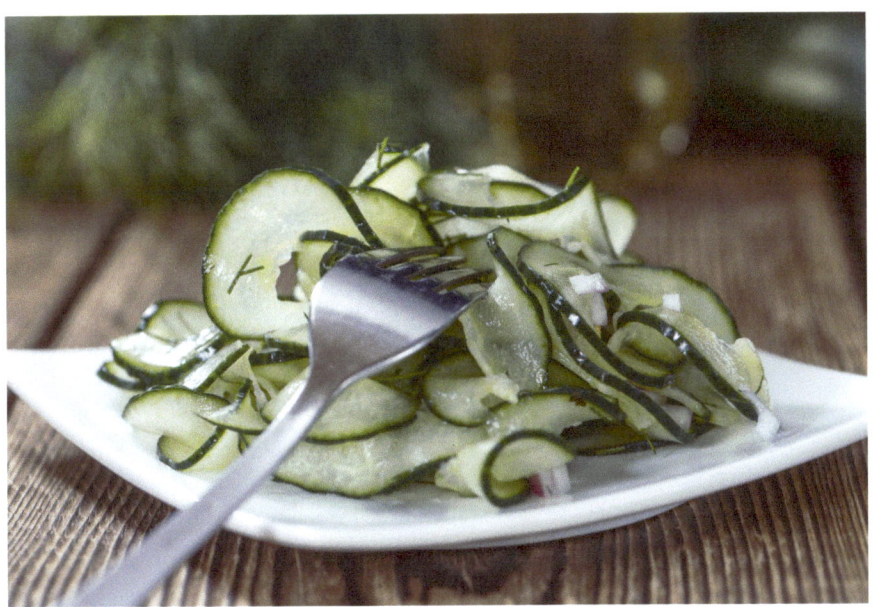

Southern Yellow Mustard Potato Salad!

Ingredients:

- 3 pounds boiled potatoes peeled and cubed
  - 6 boiled eggs chopped
  - 1 medium onion minced
  - 1/2 cup finely chopped green bell pepper
  - 1/2 cup finely chopped celery
  - 4 medium dill pickles diced
  - 3/4 cup mayonnaise
  - 1/2 cup yellow mustard
  - 1/4 Slap Ya Mamma Cajun seasoning (season to taste)
  - 1/4 teaspoon ground black pepper (optional)

Directions:

Combine all Ingredients together and mix until well-combined and creamy. Add more mayonnaise and mustard depending on tastes. Refrigerate! Keep products made with mayonnaise chilled at all time.

SOUTHERN YELLOW MUSTARD POTATO SALAD!

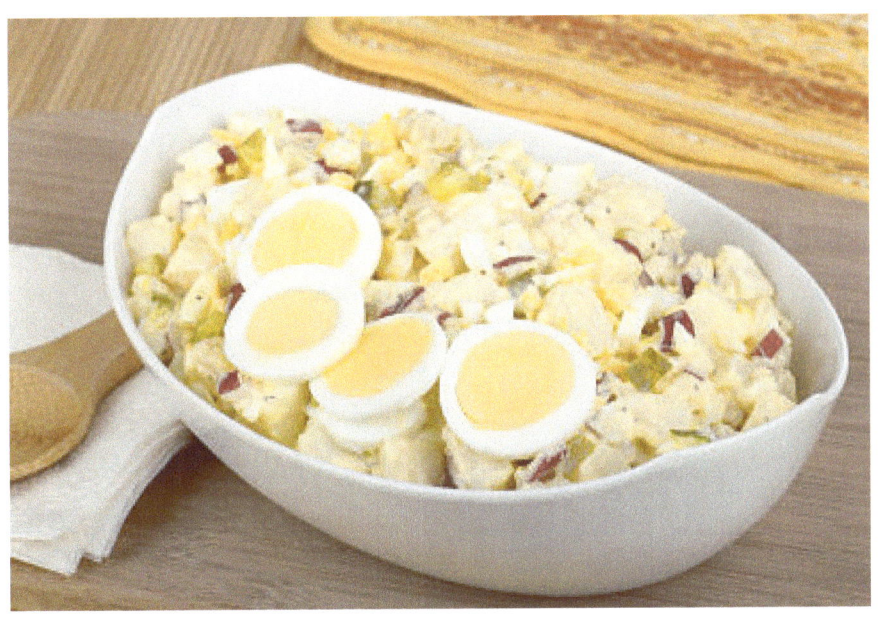

Louisiana Corn & Crab Bisque!

Ingredients:

- 2 tablespoons unsalted butter
  - 1 cup chopped onion
  - 1/2 cup chopped green bell pepper
  - 1/2 cup chopped celery
  - 1/4 cup chopped red bell pepper
  - 1 tablespoon minced garlic
  - 2 cups chicken broth
  - 1/2 cup dry white wine
  - 3/4 teaspoon dried thyme
  - 1/2 cup blond roux (1/4 cup vegetable oil and 1/4 cup flour)
  - 3½ cups heavy whipping cream
  - 1 cup cooked corn
  - 1 teaspoon Slap Ya Mamma Cajun seasoning (season to taste)
  - 1 pinch of cayenne pepper *optional
  - 1 teaspoon hot sauce
  - 1-pound lump crab-meat
  - 1 tablespoon chopped parsley
  - 1 tablespoon chopped green onion

Directions:

Heat the butter over a low to medium heat in a 4-quart sauce-pot. Add onion, green bell pepper, celery, red pepper and garlic and cook for 1 minute. Add chicken broth, white wine and thyme. Bring to boil.

In a small bowl make blond roux by combining oil and flour and stirring until a smooth paste is formed. Whip in roux until mixture begins to thicken. Whip in cream, reduce heat to a simmer and continue to cook until cream is blended in and beginning to thicken. Add salt, hot sauce and corn. Simmer 5 minutes.

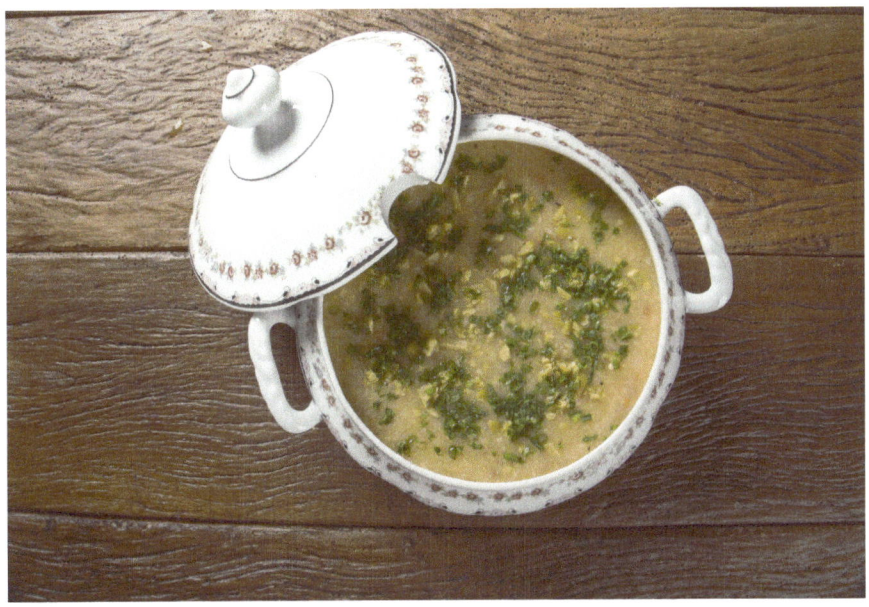

Cajun Lima Bean & Okra Soup!

Ingredients:

- 1 medium green pepper, chopped
- 1 medium onion, chopped
- 1/4 teaspoon whole cloves
- 1 tablespoon butter
- 3 cups vegetable broth
- 3 cups chopped tomatoes
- 2-1/2 cups sliced fresh or frozen okra, thawed
- 1 cup frozen Lima beans, thawed
- 1/2 cup fresh or frozen corn, thawed
- 1/2 to 1 teaspoon Slap Ya Mamma Cajun seasoning salt
- 1/4 to 1/2 teaspoon ground allspice
- 1/4 teaspoon pepper
- 1/8 teaspoon cayenne pepper to taste *optional

Directions:

- In a large saucepan, sauté the green pepper, onion and cloves in butter until vegetables are tender. Discard cloves.
- Stir in the remaining Ingredients. Bring to a boil. Reduce heat; cover and simmer for 15-20 minutes or until beans are tender.

Creole Soup!

Ingredients:

- 1-pound ground beef if you want authentic flavor use 1 14-ounce package andouille or boudin sausage
- 1 medium onion, finely chopped
- 8 cups water
- 1 can (28 ounces) diced tomatoes, undrained
- 3 cups shredded cabbage
- 3 cups cubed peeled potatoes
- 1 can (15-1/2 ounces) pork and beans
- 1 can (10-3/4 ounces) condensed tomato soup, undiluted
- 1 can (4 ounces) mushroom stems and pieces, undrained
- 1 cup sliced carrots
- 1 cup chopped green pepper
- 1 cup frozen peas
- 3 celery ribs with leaves, finely chopped
- 3 chicken bouillon cubes
- 2 tablespoons dried parsley flakes
- 1 teaspoon each Slap Ya Mamma Cajun seasoning, chili powder, Creole seasoning, pepper, crushed red pepper flakes and Italian seasoning
- Pinch of cayenne pepper to taste *optional
- 1 bay leaf

Directions:

In a soup kettle or Dutch oven, cook beef and onion over medium heat until meat is no longer pink; drain.

·Add the remaining Ingredients; bring to a boil. Reduce heat; simmer, uncovered, for 25 minutes or until vegetables are tender. Discard bay leaf before serving.

Creole Roasted Garlic Soup!

Ingredients:

- 2 tablespoons olive oil
  - 1 1/2 cups thinly sliced yellow onions
  - 1/2 cup whole peeled garlic cloves (about 16 to 20 cloves)
  - 3 bay leaves
  - 2 teaspoon salt
  - 1/2 teaspoon Slap Ya Mamma Seasoning Salt
- Black pepper
- 2 quarts white chicken stock
- 2 tablespoons minced fresh garlic
- 1 teaspoon chopped fresh basil
- 1 teaspoon chopped fresh thyme
- 2 cups torn or coarsely chopped day-old French or Italian bread
- 1/2 cup heavy cream
- 1/3 cup fresh, coarsely grated Parmesan cheese
- 1 cup spicy homemade* or prepared croutons

Directions:

- Heat the oil in a large, heavy pot over high heat and add the onions, garlic cloves, bay leaves, salt, and freshly ground black pepper to taste. Cook, stirring frequently, until the onions are caramelized, about 7 minutes. Don't let onions get too dark; they should be sweet-tasting and a rich golden-brown color.

·Stir in the stock, minced garlic, basil and thyme and bring to a boil. Reduce the heat to medium and simmer about 40 minutes. Increase the heat to high, whisk in the bread and cream and continue whisking until bread has dissolved in the soup, about 10 minutes. Whisk in the Parmesan and remove from heat. Puree soup in a food processor or blender; you may need to do this in batches depending on the size of your blender or food processor.

Serve top with toasted croutons sprinkle with Parmesan cheese

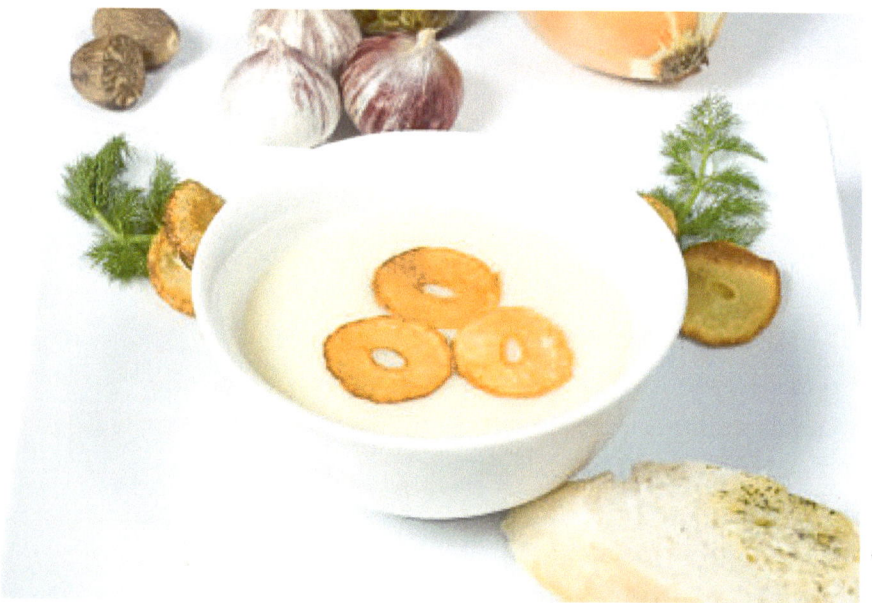

Creole Simple Tomatoes Soup!

Ingredients:

- 1/4 cup butter
  - 1/4 cup all-purpose flour
  - 1 teaspoon curry powder
  - 1/4 teaspoon onion powder
  - 1/4 teaspoon Slap Ya Mamma Cajun seasoning salt
  - Pinch cayenne pepper to taste *optional
  - 1 can (46 ounces) tomato juice
  - 1/4 cup sugar
  - Oyster crackers or croutons, optional

Directions:

- In a large saucepan, melt butter. Stir in flour, curry powder and onion powder until smooth. Gradually add tomato juice and sugar. Cook, uncovered, until thickened and heated through, about 5 minutes. If desired, serve with crackers or croutons.

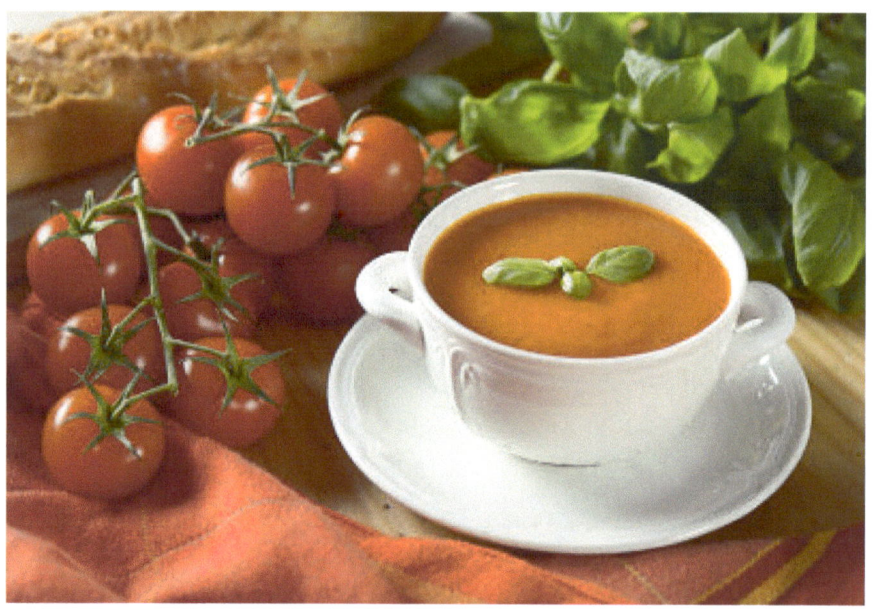

Simple Quick Tomato Soup!

Old Fashion Green Beans!

Ingredients:

- 6 bacon strips, cut into 1/2-inch pieces
- 2 pounds fresh green beans
- 3 tablespoons brown sugar
- 2 tablespoons minced onion garnish *optional
- 2 tablespoons minced parsley garnish *optional
- Pinch of Slap Ya Mamma Cajun seasoning (season to taste)
- 1/2 cup chicken broth

Directions:

- In a large skillet, cook bacon over medium heat until crisp, about 5 minutes. Add the beans, brown sugar and chicken broth pinch of Slap Ya Mamma Cajun seasoning to taste. Stir gently; bring to a boil. Reduce heat; cover and simmer for 15 minutes or until beans are crisp-tender. Remove to a serving bowl with a slotted spoon.

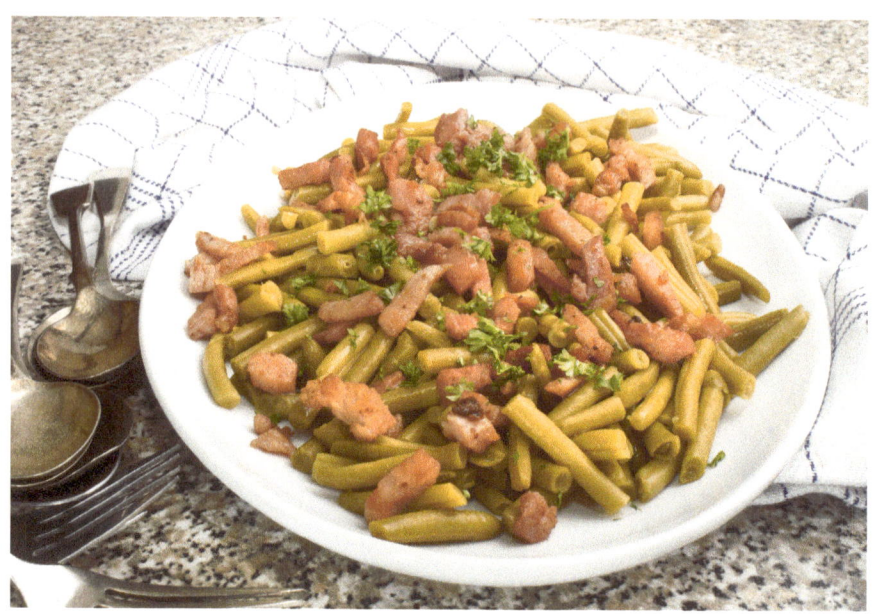

Old Fashion Green Beans!

Cajun Brussels Sprouts!

Ingredients:

- 1-1/2 pounds fresh Brussels sprouts
  - 2 teaspoons olive oil
  - 3 teaspoons butter, divided
  - 4 garlic cloves, chopped
  - 1/2 cup reduced-sodium chicken broth
  - 1/4 teaspoon Slap Ya Momma Cajun Seasoning Salt (season to taste)
  - 1/8 teaspoon pepper
  - Pinch of cayenne pepper to taste *optional*

Directions:

- Trim Brussels sprout stems. Using a paring knife, cut an "X" in the bottom of each. In a large saucepan(cast iron skillet works great), heat olive oil and 1 teaspoon butter over medium heat. Add garlic; cook and stir 1-2 minutes or until garlic begins to color. Immediately add Brussels sprouts, stirring to coat.

   Stir in broth, salt and pepper; bring to a boil. Reduce heat; simmer, covered, 8-10 minutes or until Brussels sprouts are tender. Drain. Add remaining butter; toss to coat.

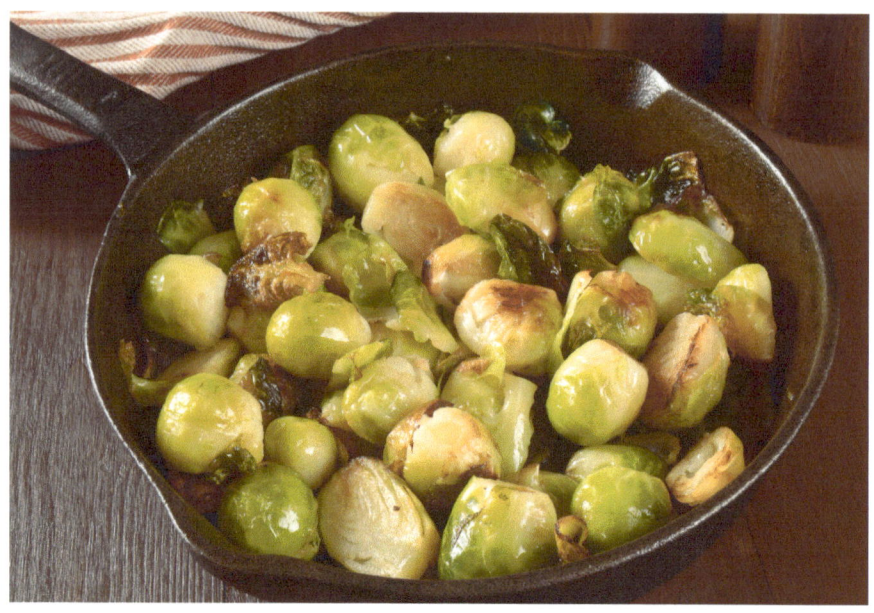

Cajun Spaghetti Supreme!

Ingredients:

- 1 package (1 pound) spaghetti, broken into 4-inch pieces
  - 1 bottle (16 ounces) zesty Italian salad dressing
  - 1 large cucumber, diced
  - 1 large tomato, seeded and diced (or 20 small cherry tomatoes cut in half)
  - 1/2 cup diced black olives
  - 2 tablespoons shredded Parmesan cheese
  - 1 teaspoon Salad Supreme Seasoning
  - 1/2 teaspoon Slap Ya Momma Cajun Seasoning Salt (season to taste)
  - Pinch of cayenne pepper to taste

Directions:

Cook spaghetti according to package directions. Drain and rinse in cold water. Place spaghetti in a large serving bowl. Add the remaining Ingredients; toss to coat. Cover and refrigerate for at least 45 minutes.

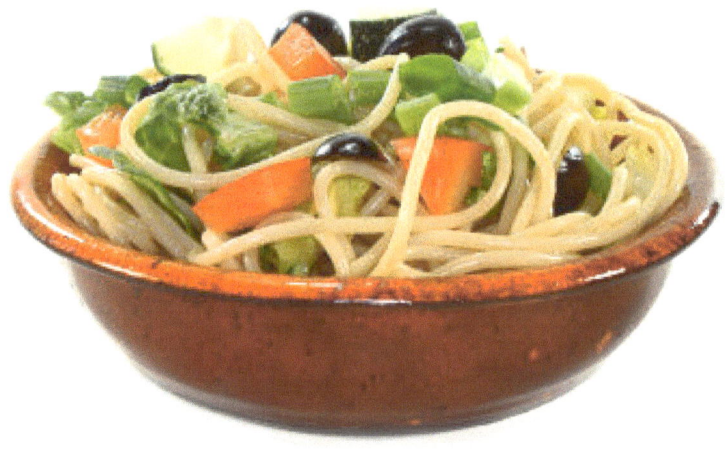

Scrumptiously Delicious **Cajun Spaghetti Supreme!**

Cajun Garlic Spaghetti!

Ingredients:

- 1 package (16 ounces) thin spaghetti
  - 4 garlic cloves, minced
  - 1/2 cup olive oil
  - 1/2 cup minced fresh parsley
  - 1/4 teaspoon of Slap Ya Momma Cajun Seasoning Salt (season to taste)
  - Pinch of cayenne pepper to taste *optional
  - Pepper to taste

Directions:

- Cook spaghetti according to package directions. Meanwhile, in a large skillet, lightly brown garlic in oil over medium heat. Drain spaghetti; add to the skillet. Sprinkle with parsley, salt and pepper; toss to coat.

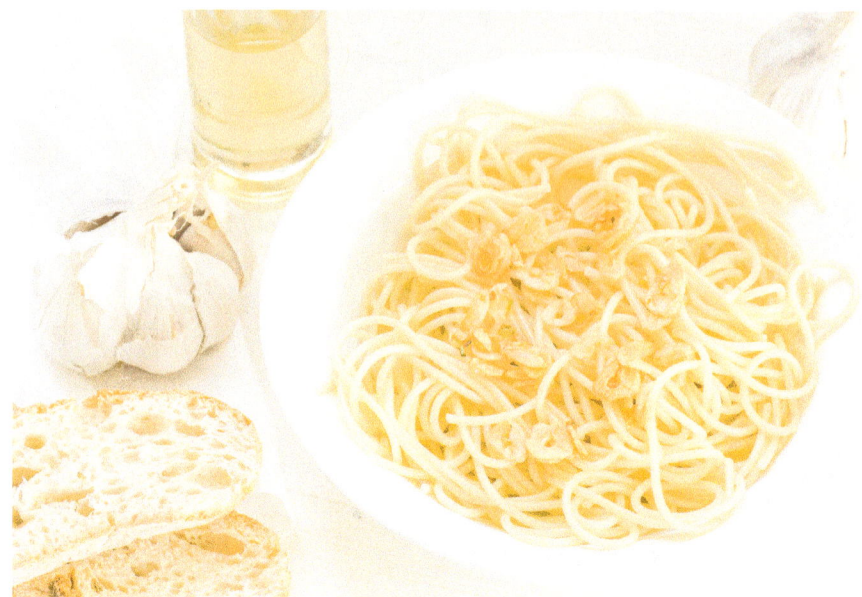

Garlic Spaghetti!

Cajun 4 Cheese Spaghetti!

Ingredients:

- 8 ounces uncooked spaghetti
  - 1/4 cup butter, cubed
  - 1 tablespoon all-purpose flour
  - 1/4 teaspoon Slap Ya Mamma seasoning salt (season to taste)
  - Pinch cayenne pepper *optional
  - 1/4 teaspoon pepper
  - 1-1/2 cups half-and-half cream
  - 1 cup shredded part-skim mozzarella cheese
  - 4 ounces fontina cheese, shredded
  - 1/2 cup shredded provolone cheese
  - 1/4 cup shredded Parmesan cheese
  - 2 tablespoons minced fresh parsley

Directions:

- Cook spaghetti according to package directions. Meanwhile, in a large saucepan, melt butter. Stir in the flour, salt and pepper until smooth. Gradually stir in cream. Bring to a boil; cook and stir for 2 minutes or until thickened. Remove from the heat; stir in all cheeses until melted.
  - Drain spaghetti; toss with cheese sauce and garnish with parsley.

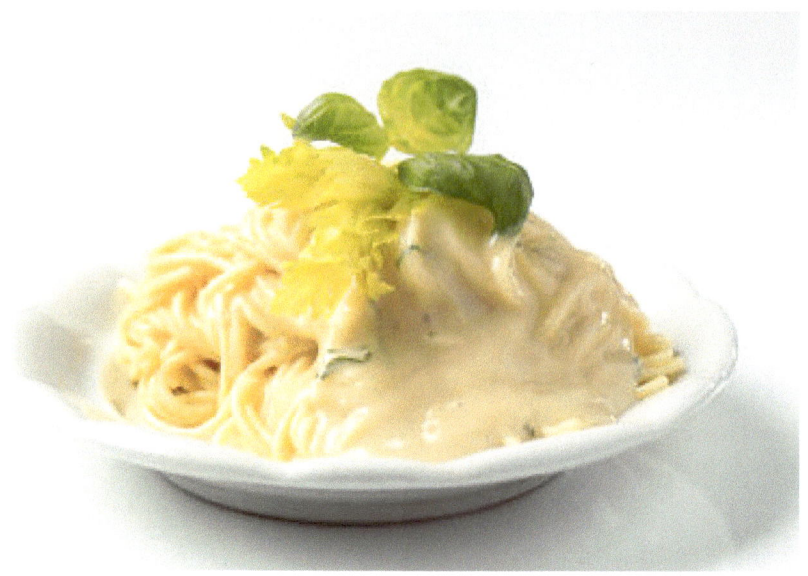

Authentic Cajun Homemade Macaroni & Cheese!

Ingredients:

- 1 tablespoon butter
  - 1 Andouille sausage, sliced
  - 1/3 cup finely diced onion
  - 2 tablespoons finely diced red bell pepper
  - 1 cup cooked crawfish tails
  - 8 ounces mini penne or elbow pasta, cooked al dente
  - 2 eggs, lightly beaten
  - 2/3 cup milk
  - 1/4 teaspoon paprika
  - 1/8 teaspoon garlic powder
  - 1/4 teaspoon ground white pepper
  - 1 teaspoons Slap Ya Mamma Cajun seasoning (season to taste)
  - Pinch of cayenne pepper *optional
  - 1 1/2 cups grated sharp cheddar cheese
  - 1 cup shredded white cheddar
  - 1 cup shredded Mozzarella cheese
  - 1/2 cup shredded Parmesan
  - 1/2 cup crushed Ritz crackers

Directions:

·Preheat oven to 350 degrees. Coat a 2-quart baking dish with cooking spray.

·Melt butter in a sauté pan. Add Andouille sausage and sauté for 2 minutes. Add onion, red bell pepper, and crawfish. Sauté 2 minutes and remove from heat.

·Place cooked pasta in a large bowl. Whisk together eggs and milk and pour in bowl with pasta.

·Add spices and salt to pasta bowl along with crawfish mixture.

·Mix cheeses in a medium bowl and set aside 1/2 cup of cheese. Add the rest of the cheese to the pasta. Mix together well and pour into prepared dish.

·Sprinkle cracker crumbs and reserved 1/2 cup cheese on top.

·Cover dish with aluminum foil and bake 15 minutes. Remove foil and bake uncovered for 5 minutes.

**This recipe is great for just plain old-fashioned macaroni and cheese also, just leave out the Andouille sausage and cooked crawfish tails.

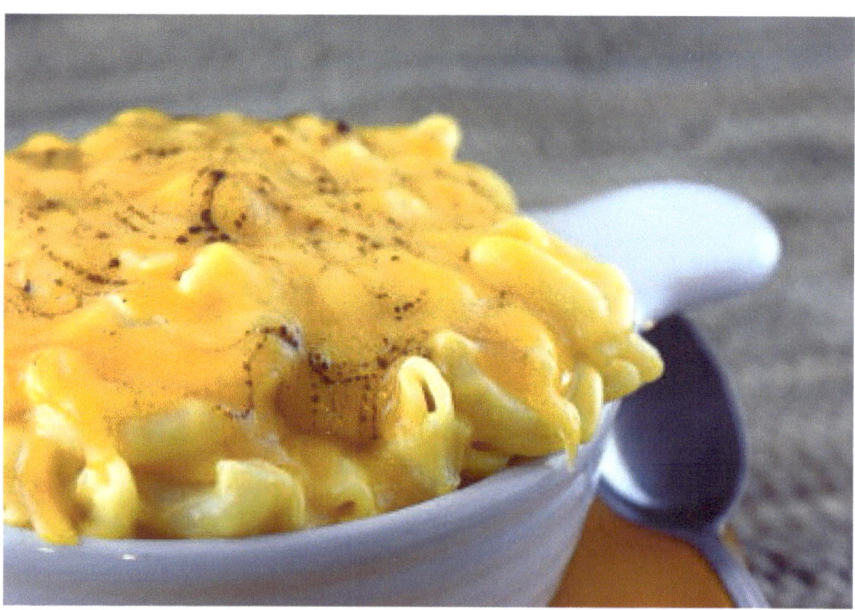

Cajun Chicken Breast!

Ingredients:

- 1/4 cup all-purpose flour
  - 1/2 teaspoon Slap Ya Momma Seasoning Salt
  - Pinch of cayenne pepper to taste *optional
  - 1/2 teaspoon pepper
  - 4 boneless skinless chicken breast halves (4 ounces each)
  - 1/4 cup butter, cubed (use slightly salted)
  - 1/4 cup white wine or chicken broth
  - 1 tablespoon lemon juice
  - Fresh parsley garnish , optional

Directions:

In a shallow bowl, mix flour, salt and pepper. Pound chicken breasts with a meat mallet to 1/2-in. thickness. Dip chicken in flour mixture to coat lightly both sides; shake off excess.

    In a large skillet, heat butter over medium heat. Brown chicken on both sides. Add wine; bring to a boil. Reduce heat; simmer, uncovered, until chicken is no longer pink, 12-15 minutes. Drizzle with lemon juice. If desired, sprinkle with parsley.

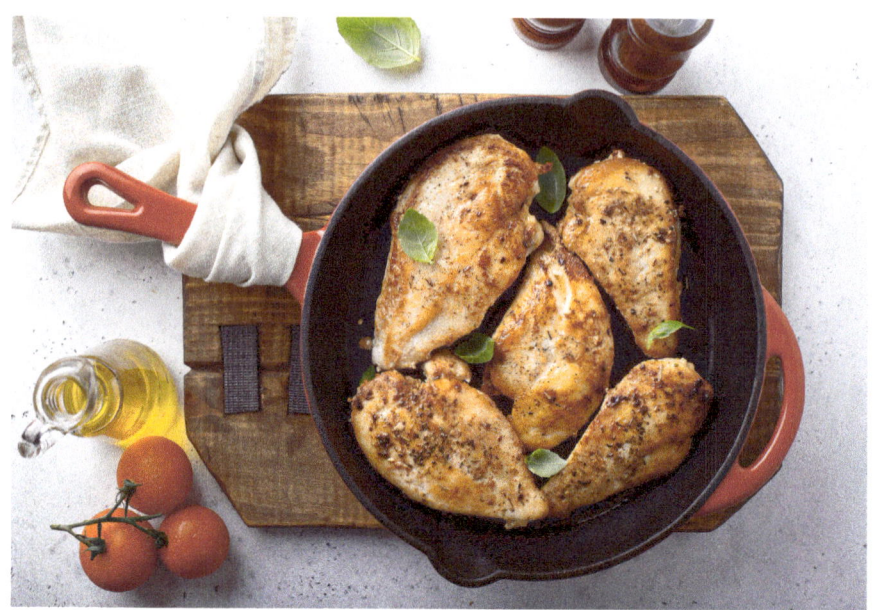

Cajun Fried Chicken!

Cajun Fried Chicken

Ingredients:

- 2 cups butter milk
  - 2 tablespoons Slap Ya Mamma Cajun seasoning
  - ¼ teaspoon ground pepper
  - ¼ teaspoon white pepper or black pepper
  - Pinch of cayenne pepper
  - 8 boneless skinless chicken breast halves (4 ounces each)
  - 4 boneless skinless chicken thighs (about 1 pound), halved
  - 1-1/4 cups all-purpose flour
  - 1/2 teaspoon lemon-pepper seasoning
  - 1/2 teaspoon garlic salt
  - ½ teaspoon garlic powder *optional
  - ½ teaspoon onion powder*optional
  - 5 dashes of Louisiana Hot Sauce
  - Oil for frying
  - *note if you use bone in chicken may need extra cook time*

Directions:

In a large bowl, combine buttermilk and 1 tablespoon Slap Ya Mamma Cajun seasoning; ground pepper, cayenne pepper, garlic powder, onion power, hot sauce and mix well and then add chicken. Cover and refrigerate for at least 2 hours.

In a large shallow dish, combine the flour, 1 tablespoon of Slap Ya Mamma Cajun seasoning, garlic salt and remaining Cajun seasoning, any pepper left add all to flour mixture. Next drain chicken and discard milk mixture. Next place or dip chicken in flour mixture and turn to coat.

In a skillet, heat 1/4 in. of oil; fry chicken in batches until golden brown and juices run clear, 7-8 minutes. Drain on paper towel.

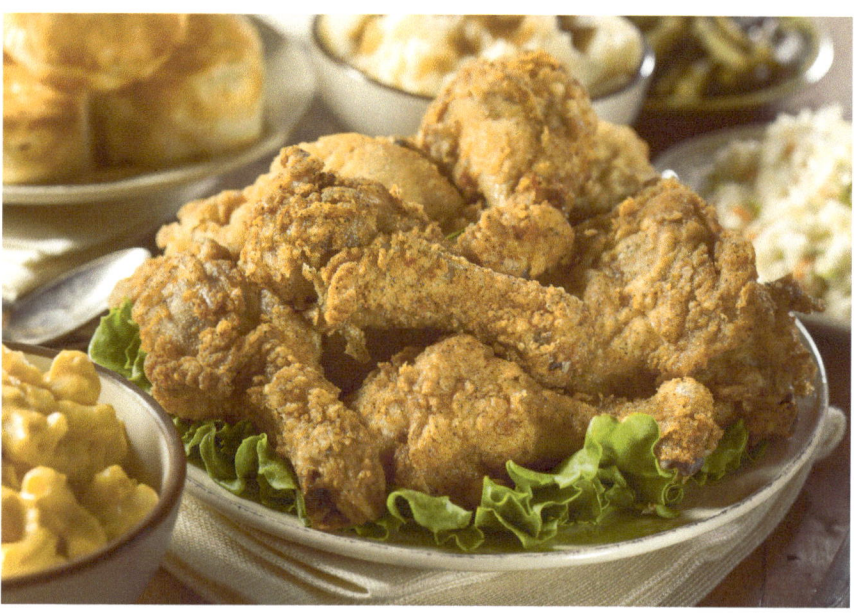

Cajun Pan Seared Salmon!

Ingredients:

- 4 salmon fillets (6 ounces each)
  - 1 teaspoon Slap Ya Mamma Cajun seasoning
  - 1/4 teaspoon black pepper
  - 1/2 cup reduced-fat plain yogurt
  - 1/4 cup reduced-fat mayonnaise
  - 1/4 cup finely chopped cucumber
  - 1 teaspoon snipped fresh dill
  - 1 tablespoon canola oil

Directions:

- In a large skillet, heat oil over medium-high heat. Sprinkle salmon with Slap Ya Mamma Cajun seasoning and pepper. Place in skillet, skin side down. Reduce heat to medium. Cook until fish just begins to flake easily with a fork, about 5 minutes on each side.
  - Meanwhile, in a small bowl, combine yogurt, mayonnaise, cucumber and dill. Serve with salmon.
    - ***This recipe can be used with halibut, swordfish, or tuna.***

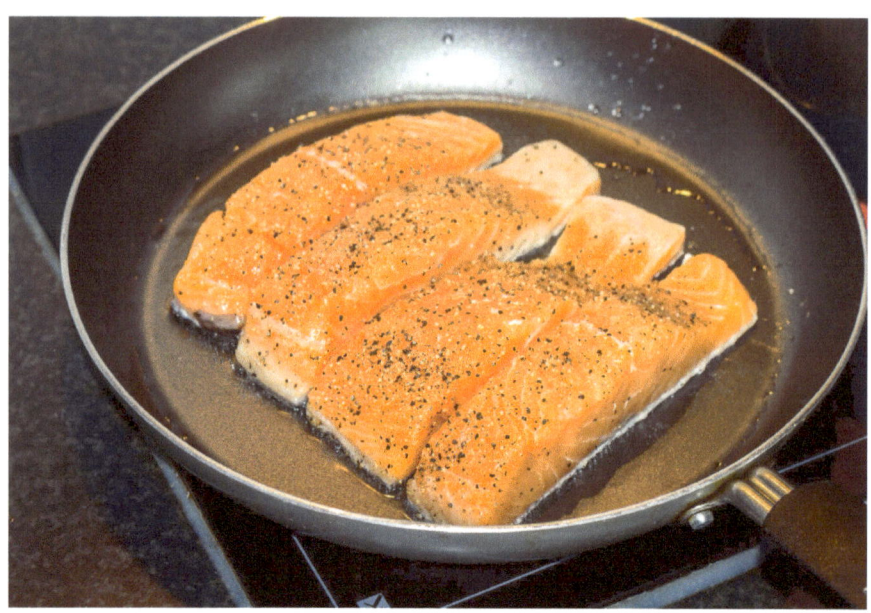

*This recipe can be used with halibut, swordfish, or tuna.

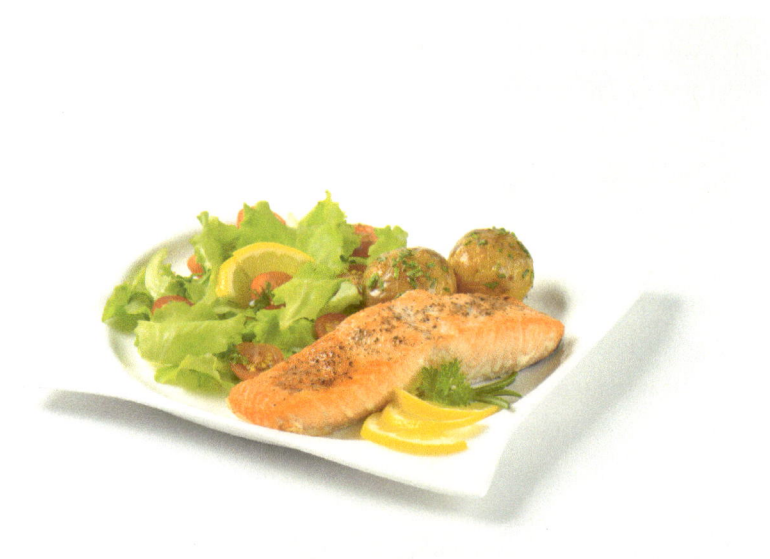

Cajun Shrimp Sandwich!

* Makes An Excellent Appetizer*

Ingredients:

·1 teaspoon kosher salt

·12 ounces medium shrimp (peeled and *devein*) (Check Wal-Mart Supermarket for great low price...less than $10.00 a bag on already clean shrimp.)

·1 1/2 teaspoons Slap Ya Mamma Cajun seasoning (see note at end)

·2 teaspoons lemon juice (or to taste)

·1/3 cup mayonnaise

·1/4 teaspoon Worcestershire sauce

·1 to 2 ribs celery, chopped (about 1/2 cup)

·1 to 2 scallions, chopped (about 1/3 cup)

·2 sandwich rolls, hoagie rolls, or large hamburger buns (split and toasted)

·3/4 cup shredded iceberg or romaine lettuce

·Sliced large tomatoes

Directions:

Gather the Ingredients.

Add the kosher salt to a quart or so of water in a medium pot.

Bring just to a simmer and add the shrimp. Stir and cook for 1 to 2 minutes (depending on the size of the shrimp); they should be pink and barely translucent.

Drain and rinse briefly under cool water. Drain thoroughly.

Place the shrimp in a small bowl and add 1/2 teaspoon of the and 1 teaspoon of the lemon juice.

Toss to coat and place in the refrigerator for 20 minutes or so to cool completely.

Whisk the remaining Slap Yo Mamma seasoning, remaining lemon juice, mayonnaise, and Worcestershire sauce together in a medium-size bowl.

When the shrimp are cool, add them along with the celery and scallions to the dressing and toss gently to coat. Adjust seasoning, adding more lemon juice and salt if necessary.

Serve on toasted rolls or buns with shredded lettuce. To make assembly and eating less messy, scoop out part of the inside

Optional can use this recipe for oysters too! Just substitute the shrimp for oysters. If you want shrimp or oysters fried. See Fried Catfish recipe

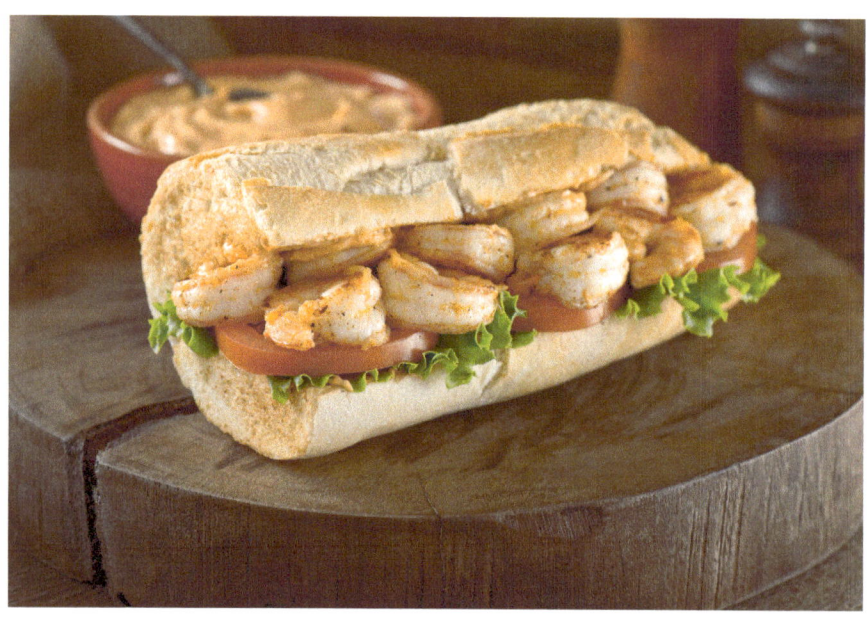

Spicy Cajun Shrimp Sandwich W/Chipotle Avocado...

Spicy Cajun Shrimp Sandwich W/Chipotle Avocado Mayonnaise

Ingredients:

- 1/2 teaspoon cumin
- 1/2 teaspoon garlic powder
- 1/4 teaspoon kosher salt
- 1/4 teaspoon chili powder
- ¼ teaspoon Slap Ya Mamma Cajun seasoning
- 2 teaspoons olive oil
- 1/2-pound medium shrimp (about 20 shrimp) peeled and deveined Check Wal-Mart Supermarket for great low price...less than $10.00 a bag.)
- 1 avocado, pitted and diced
- 1/2 cup mayonnaise
- 1 chipotle pepper
- Juice of 1 lime
- 1/4 teaspoon kosher salt
- 2 French rolls
- 4 romaine lettuce leaves

Directions:

Combine cumin, garlic powder, 1/4 teaspoon kosher salt ¼ teaspoon Slap Ya Mamma Cajun seasoning, chili powder and olive oil together in a bowl. Place shrimp in the bowl and toss to coat.

Combine avocado, mayonnaise, chipotle pepper, lime juice and 1/4 teaspoon kosher salt in a food processor. Pulse until smooth.

Place shrimp in a skillet over medium heat. Cook until pink and cooked through, about 5 minutes.

Toast rolls, if desired. Spread chipotle avocado mayonnaise on the roll. Place lettuce leaves on the bottom half of the roll and place 10 shrimp on each sandwich.

Serve.

Cajun Catfish Tacos Deep Fried or Oven Baked

Ingredients:

1-pound skinless catfish fillets, cut into 16 pieces

3/4 cup whole buttermilk

1/2 cup fine yellow cornmeal

1/2 cup panko (Japanese-style breadcrumbs) *If you don't have panko. Substitutions for panko. Try toasted shredded bread, cracker crumbs, crushed Melba toasts, matzo meal, crushed tortilla chips, crushed dry stuffing mix, crushed pretzels, crushed cornflakes, or crushed potato chips*

2 tablespoons Slap Ya Mamma Cajun seasoning

3/4 teaspoon kosher salt, divided

1/4 cup mayonnaise

2 tablespoons fresh lime juice (from 1 lime)

1/4 teaspoon black pepper

2 cups shredded green cabbage (from 1 small cabbage)

8 (6-inch) yellow corn tortillas, warmed

2 radishes, cut into matchsticks (1/4 cup)

1 ripe avocado, thinly sliced

2 tablespoons fresh cilantro leaves

2 tablespoons minced fresh chives

Lime wedges

Louisiana Hot sauce (Or Franks Hot sauce or Crystals Hot sauce)

Directions:

Steps for Baking & or Frying Catfish Listed below...

Step 1

Preheat oven to 450°F with oven rack 6 inches from heat. Combine catfish and buttermilk in a medium bowl; cover and chill 20 minutes or up to 1 hour

Step 2 If you want to Bake Catfish follow here...

Whisk together cornmeal, panko, Cajun seasoning, and 1/4 teaspoon of the salt in a shallow dish. Drain catfish; discard buttermilk. Working in batches, dredge fish in cornmeal mixture. Place fish on a wire rack set inside a rimmed baking sheet. Bake in preheated oven until it's golden brown and flakes with a fork, 20 to 25 minutes.

Deep Frying Fish Instructions:

**If you want to deep fry catfish have oil for frying and a large skillet.

Heat 1/4 in. of oil in a large skillet; fry fish over medium-high heat for 3-4 minutes on each side or until fish flakes easily with a fork. Drain on a paper towel.

Step 3

Meanwhile, whisk together mayonnaise, lime juice, pepper, and remaining 1/2 teaspoon salt in a medium bowl. Add cabbage; toss to coat.

Step 4

Place 2 pieces of catfish in each tortilla. Top with cabbage mixture, radishes, avocado, cilantro, and chives. Serve with lime wedges and hot sauce.

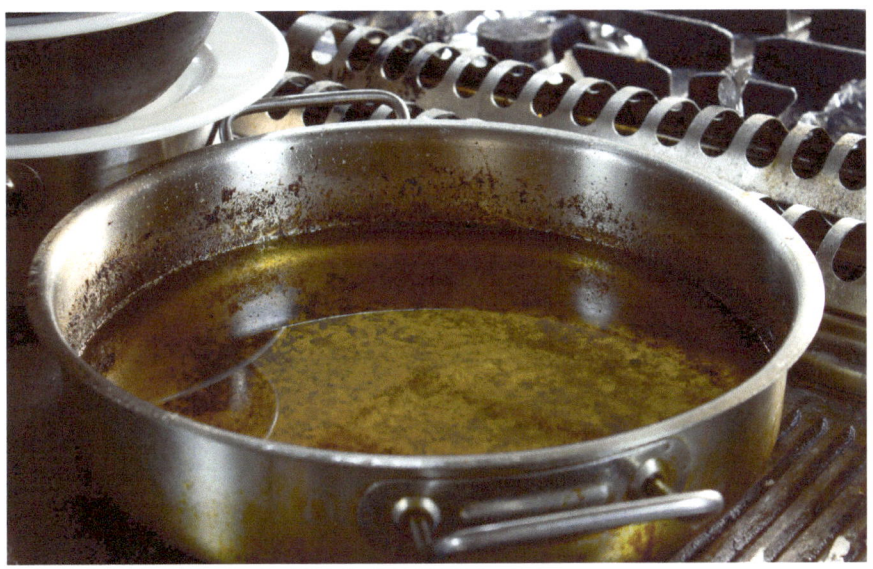

Heat oil for frying in a large pot...If deep frying catfish.

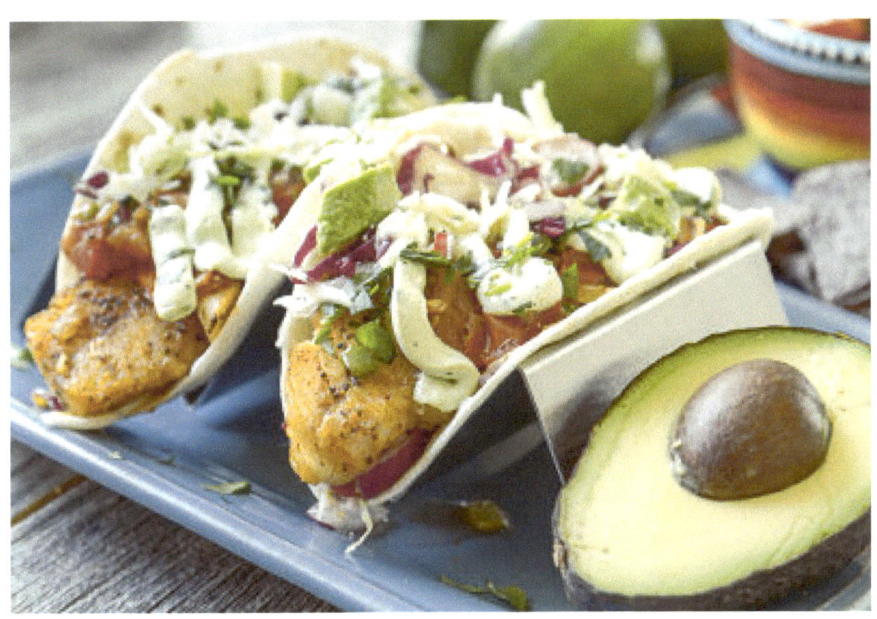

Deep Fried or Baked Catfish Tacos tastes delicious!

Fried Cajun Catfish!

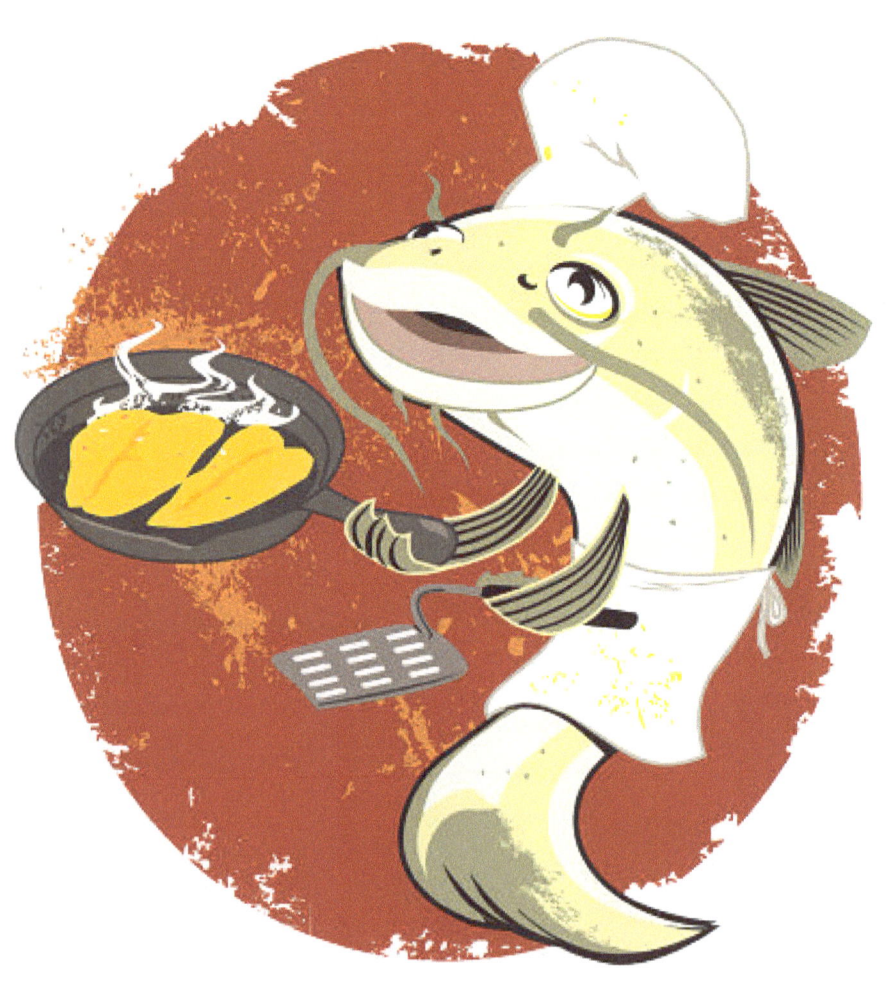

FRIED CAJUN CATFISH!

Cast iron skillet fries the best, but deep-dish stainless steel is good too...

Ingredients:

- Catfish (nugget or fillet)
  - 2 cups yellow cornmeal
  - 2 tbsp salt
  - (optional replace salt with Slap Ya Mamma Cajun seasoning)
  - 2 tbsp pepper
  - 2 tbsp cayenne pepper
  - 2 tbsp onion powder
  - 2 tbsp garlic powder
  - 2 tbsp paprika
- Cooking oil

Optional Steps ½ cup Louisiana Hot Sauce

½ cup apple cider vinegar

Directions:

Preheat cooking oil in frying pan to 375 degrees (can test with a few drops of cornmeal should hear a good sizzling sound)

In a large bowl mix cornmeal and all seasonings·In a separate bowl combine Louisiana Hot Sauce and apple cider vinegar
   Coat each piece of fish in Hot Sauce and vinegar mixture
   Next drench/coat each piece of fish well with cornmeal breading
   Place fish a few pieces at a time in the frying pan
   Cook for 4 minutes to five minutes on both sides or to your liking, should be a nice golden brown crispy looking.
   *** You can also use the steps her for frying Large Shrimp or Oysters, however, watch cooking time, as Shrimp and Oysters are smaller than Fish filet.**

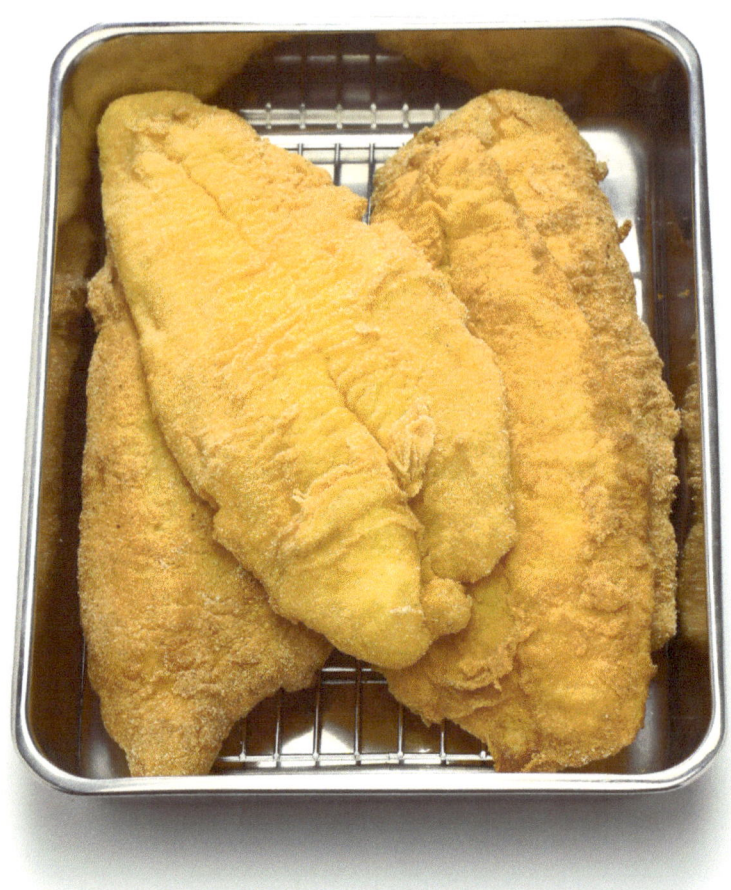

Deep Fried Catfish!

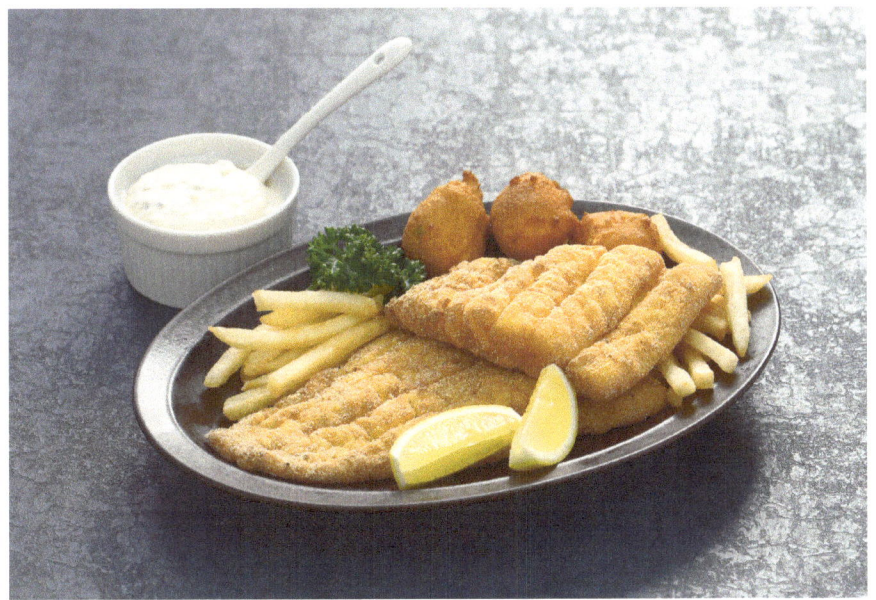

Catfish dinner suggestion.

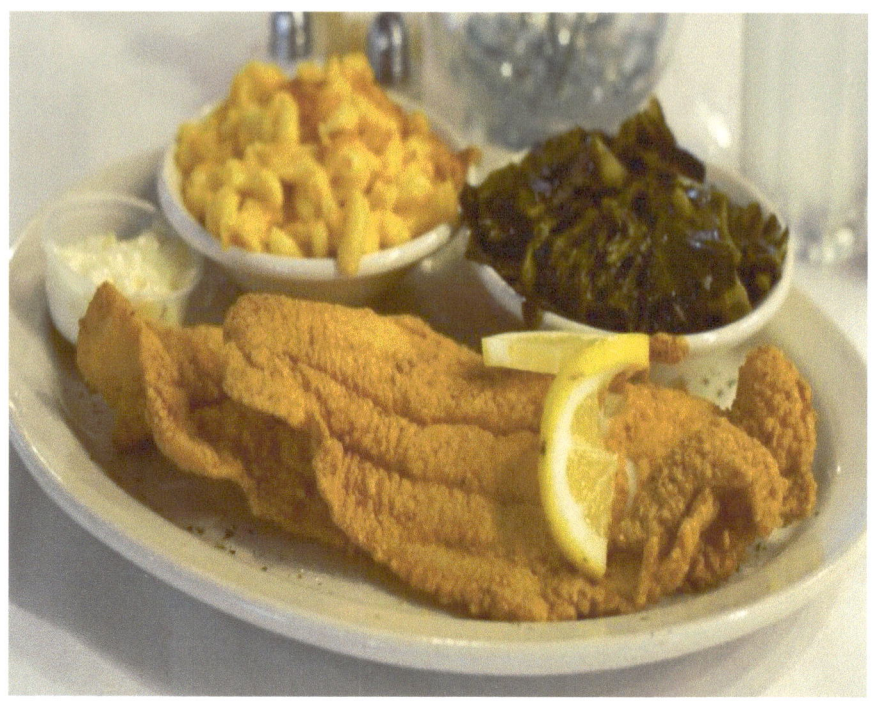

Soul Food Catfish Dinner with Collard Greens and Macaroni and Cheese

Cajun Buttery Steak Bites!

Ingredients:

Use a 23 oz cut of steak, which can be Sirloin, Rump, New York Strip, Porterhouse or Rib-eye. Next cut into 2-inch cubes
- 1-2 tablespoons canola oil, divided
- 1/4 cup butter
- 4 cloves garlic finely chopped
- 3 tablespoons of Slap Ya Mamma Cajun seasoning.

Directions:

Toss steak pieces in Slap Ya Mamma Cajun seasoning.
- Heat skillet or pan to just smoking hot. (This is the secret to the best sear)
- For medium steak bites, sear for two minutes each side. For well-done bites, sear 3-4 minutes each side. Then set aside.
- Once the steak is cooked to your liking, reduce the heat and add butter and garlic to the hot pan.
- Take the pan off the heat and toss your steak bites in the garlic butter.
- Serve.

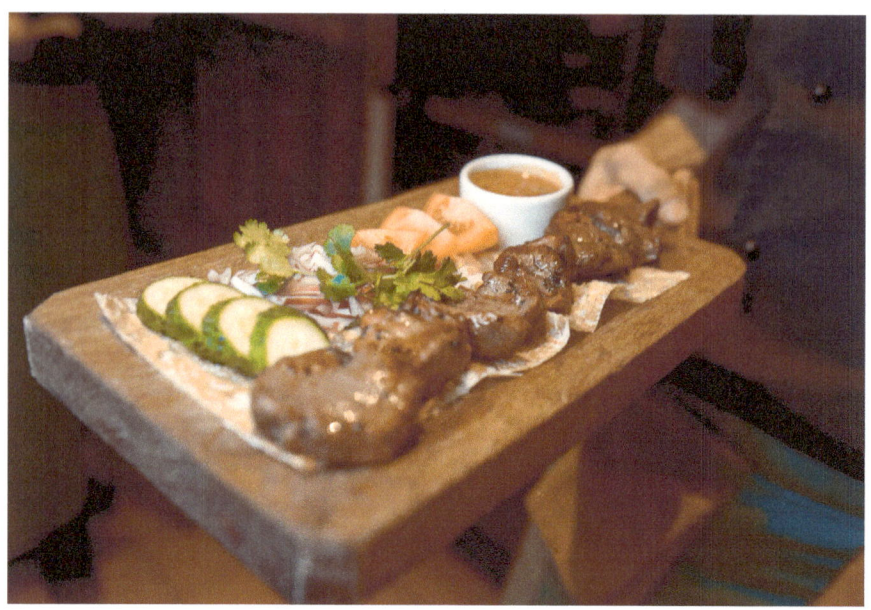

Cajun Buttery Steak Bites!

Cajun Style Beef Tips & Rice!

Ingredients:

- 3 tablespoons vegetable oil
  - 1 onion, chopped
  - 2 pounds cubed beef stew meat
  - 2 cups water
  - 1/4 cup soy sauce
  - 1/4 cup Worcestershire sauce
  - 1 teaspoon garlic powder
  - 1 teaspoon onion powder
  - 1 teaspoon Slap Ya Mamma Cajun seasoning
  - 1 teaspoon ground black pepper
  - 1 (.75 ounce) packet dry brown gravy mix
  - 1 cup water

Directions:

1. In a large skillet heat oil over high heat. Sauté the onion until almost translucent.

2. Season stew meat with ½ teaspoon each of the garlic powder, onion powder, and Slap Ya Mamma Cajun season. Add the stew meat and cook on high heat until meat is browned on all sides; about 3 to 5 minutes.

3. Pour 2 cups water, soy sauce, and Worcestershire sauce into the skillet.

Stir in remaining ½ teaspoon of garlic powder, onion powder, Slap Ya Mamma Cajun seasoning and the black pepper. Bring to a boil and reduce heat. Cover and simmer for 1 1/2 to 2 hours.

4.Meanwhile combine the gravy mix with 1 cup water. Mix thoroughly and stir into the meat mixture. Bring to a boil stirring frequently until slightly thickened.

For Rice Follow These Steps

1.Boil water and add salt. After your rinse your rise, pour water (for every cup of **rice**, use 1¾ cups of water) into a large saucepan with a tight-fitting lid. ...

2. Pour in rice. Add the rice to the boiling water.
3. Stir once, or just enough to separate the rice. ...
4. Cover the pot and simmer. ...
5. Fluff rice with a fork.

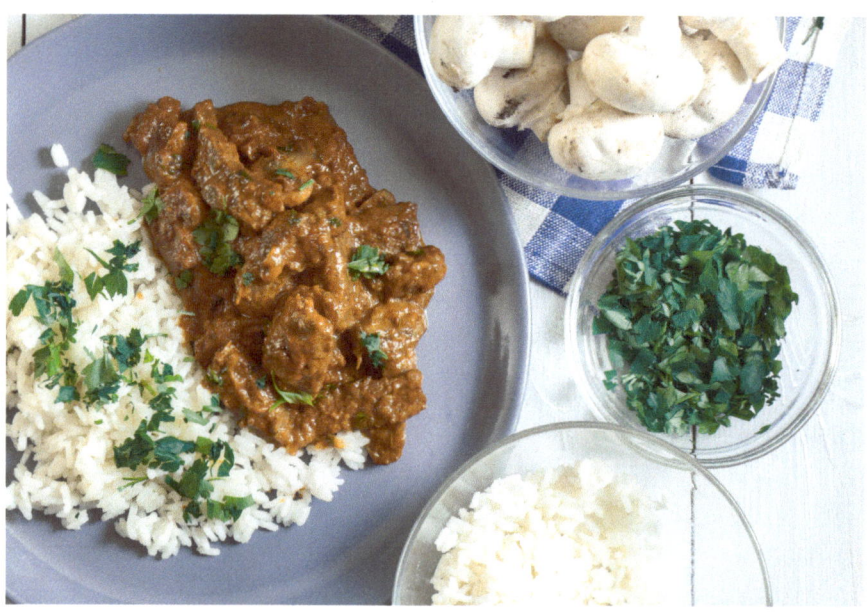

Cajun Bone-In Rib Eye Steaks

Ingredients:

- 2 tablespoons + 1 teaspoon black pepper
- 2 tablespoons + 1 teaspoon cayenne pepper
- 2 tablespoons + 1 teaspoon white ground pepper
- 2 tablespoons + 1 teaspoons paprika
- 1 tablespoon + 1 teaspoon garlic powder
- 1 tablespoon + 1 teaspoon chili powder
- 2 teaspoons basil, dried
- 1 tablespoon + 1 teaspoon kosher salt
- 1 tablespoon + 1 teaspoon ground cumin
- 2 teaspoons thyme, dried, whole

Cajun Marinade:

- 1 cup salad oil
- 1/2 cup Cajun Spice Rub
- 1/2 Spanish onion

To Marinate Steaks:

- 1/2 cup Cajun spice
- 1 cup Cajun Marinade oil
- 1/2 Spanish onion
- 4 Rib Eye steaks

Directions:

•Combine all Ingredients for the spicy rub, mix well. Set aside.

•If you do not want to marinade for a couple of hours, you can simply rub steaks generously with Cajun Spice Rub on both sides and cook.

If Using Marinate:

• Combine all Ingredients for the spicy rub. Place Ingredients into stock pot and simmer for one hour.

•Strain through a mesh fine hole strainer.

•Store in a plastic container.

•To Marinate Steaks: Use a fork to pierce the meat, pressing the rub into the steak.

•Slice onions.

•Place the steaks and oil in a plastic container just large enough to hold them.

•Add oil to cover the steaks

•Marinate in a refrigerator for two days.

•For Cooking: Season steaks with a bit of salt.

Grill or broil to desired temperature.

•Finish with a bit of Cajun oil before serving.

CAJUN BONE-IN RIB EYE STEAKS

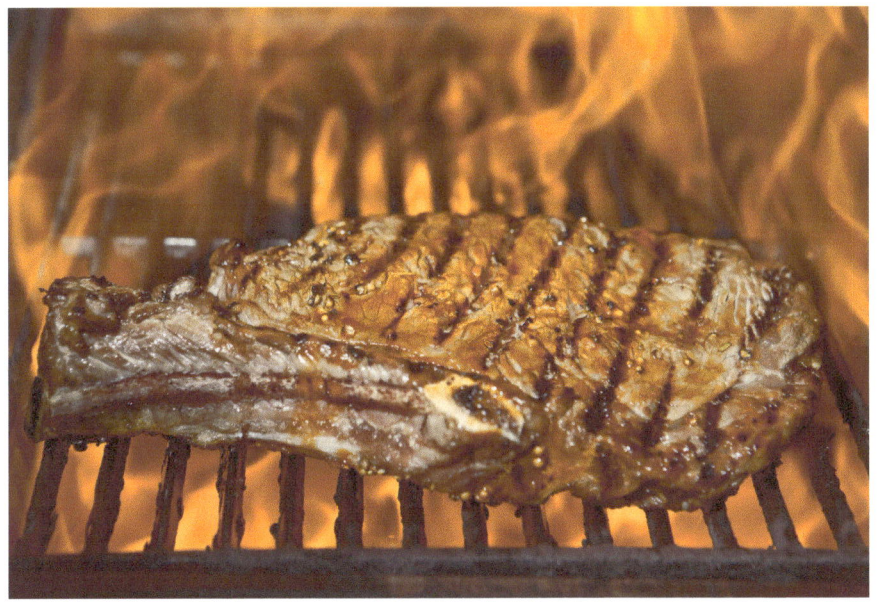

This recipe works great with rib-eye, T-bone, and Porterhouse steaks too.

Create Your own Rub: Cajun Seasoning!

Homemade Mild Cajun Seasoning:

Ingredients:

- 1 tablespoon mild paprika
  - 1 1/2 teaspoons salt
  - 1 1/2 teaspoons garlic powder
  - 1 teaspoon onion powder
  - 1 teaspoon chili powder, add more if you like heat
  - 3/4 teaspoon dried thyme
  - 1/2 teaspoon dried oregano
  - 1 1/2 teaspoon brown sugar KETO: use brown sugar substitute
  - 1/2-3/4 teaspoon cayenne pepper, add more if you like heat
  - 1/4 teaspoon cracked

Directions:

Combine all ingredients, making sure brown sugar is evenly distributed. Store in an airtight container for up to 6 months.

Notes:
Rubs consist of two components, salty and sweet. You can build on those components with other flavors and spices, but those are the building blocks to properly season meat.

Keep your dry homemade rubs and spices tightly covered and store them in a cool, dry place. Whole spices stay fresh for up to 2 years while ground spices have a 6-month shelf life. Store red spices, such as paprika and red pepper, in the refrigerator. They will hold their color and keep their flavor longer.

Apply your dry rub about an hour before you add your meat to the barbecue. Large roasts, whole poultry and big cuts of meat like brisket can benefit from being rubbed the night before. The salt and sugar will draw out the moisture from the meat and all the flavors of the spices can mellow and marinate on the surface.

* * *

Cajun Spicy Rub for Pork or Beef:

Ingredient:

- 2 tablespoons + 1 teaspoon black pepper
  - 2 tablespoons + 1 teaspoon cayenne pepper
  - 2 tablespoons + 1 teaspoon white ground pepper
  - 2 tablespoons + 1 teaspoons paprika
  - 1 tablespoon + 1 teaspoon garlic powder
  - 1 tablespoon + 1 teaspoon chili powder
  - 2 teaspoons basil, dried
  - 1 tablespoon + 1 teaspoon kosher salt
  - 1 tablespoon + 1 teaspoon ground cumin
  - 2 teaspoons thyme, dried, whole

Directions:

Combine all ingredients, making sure brown sugar is evenly distributed. Store in an airtight container for up to 6 months.

Notes:

Rubs consist of two components, salty and sweet. You can build on those components with other flavors and spices, but those are the building blocks to properly season meat.

Keep your dry homemade rubs and spices tightly covered and store them in a cool, dry place. Whole spices stay fresh for up to 2 years while ground spices have a 6-month shelf life. Store red spices, such as paprika and red pepper, in the refrigerator. They will hold their color and keep their flavor longer.

Apply your dry rub about an hour before you add your meat to the barbecue. Large roasts, whole poultry and big cuts of meat like brisket can benefit from being rubbed the night before. The salt and sugar will draw out the moisture from the meat and all the flavors of the spices can mellow and marinate on the surface.

CREATE YOUR OWN RUB: CAJUN SEASONING!

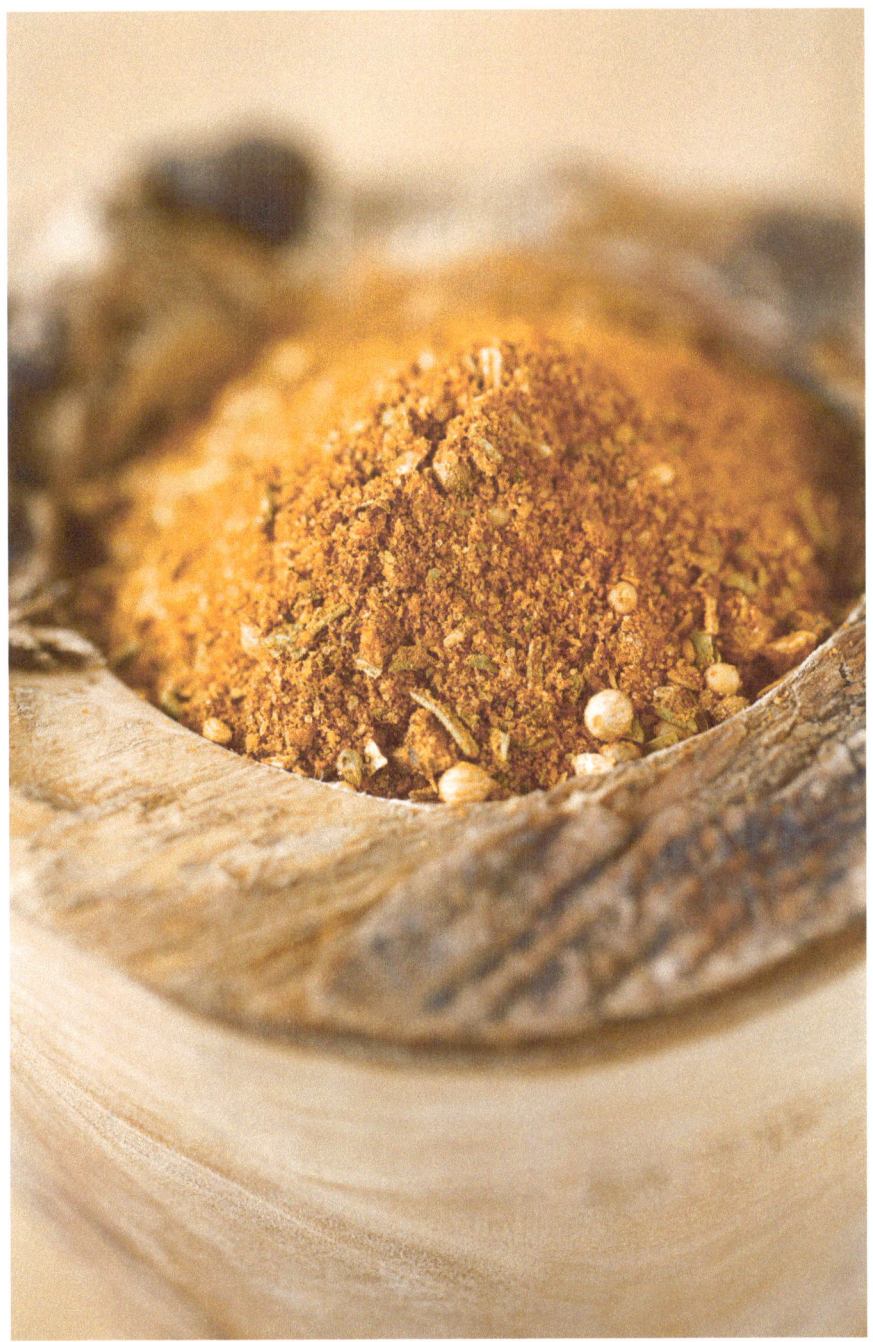

Create your own homemade rub!

Cajun Pork Chops!

Ingredients:

- 1 tsp fresh cracked black pepper
- 1 tsp red pepper
- ½ tsp Slap Ya Momma Cajun seasonings
- 1 tsp white pepper
- 4 center cut pork chops
- 1 tbs butter
- 1 small can of diced tomatoes
- 2 cloves garlic, sliced
- 1 small onion, diced
- 1 tbs fresh parsley, chopped

Directions:

- Combine black pepper, white pepper and red pepper. Mix well.
- Sprinkle on both sides of the chops.
- In a large sauté pan add the butter using medium high heat and add the chops.
- Lower the heat to medium and saute the chops for about 5 minutes, turning halfway through cooking.
- Add the tomatoes, garlic and onion, partially cover and cook for another 10 minutes or until pork is tender.

- Remove pork with a slotted spoon and add to a serving dish.
- Continue to cook sauce until thickened.

Spoon sauce over pork and serve.

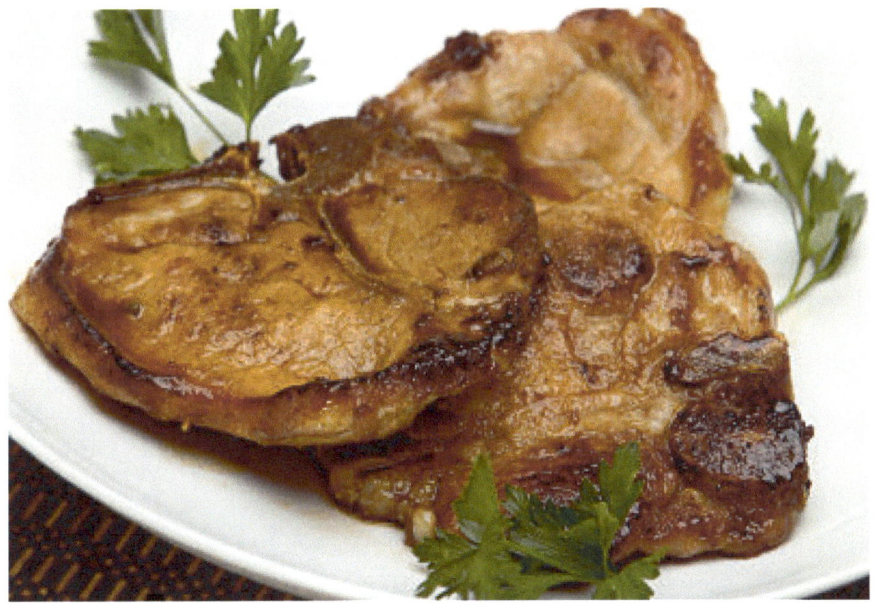

Cajun Style Roast Pork!

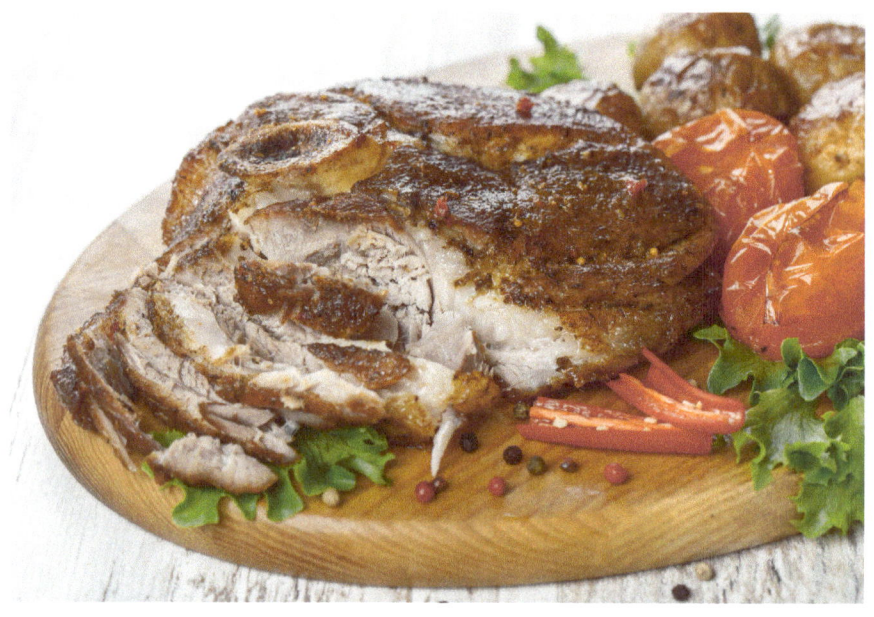

Pork Roast!

Serves 8 to 10

Ingredient:

1 (8 lb.) bone-in pork shoulder, with most of the fat trimmed 2 tablespoons Slap Ya Mamma Cajun Seasoning, Black pepper to taste.

2 yellow onions, quartered , 3 medium potatoes, 2 stalks of chopped celery, 6 baby carrots, halved lengthwise (or 4 carrots, quartered) 2 large sweet red peppers halved, 8 ounces of mushrooms cleaned and cut in half, 1 1/2 bunches thyme 1 bunch sage.

Directions:

1. Spread Slap Ya Mamma Cajun seasoning mix over pork roast until completely covered. 2. Wrap roast in plastic wrap and refrigerate for at least 4 hours, and up to 24 hours.

3. **Preheat oven to 450°F.**

4. Arrange carrots, potatoes, chopped celery, sweet red peppers, mushrooms, thyme, and sage into the bottom of a roasting pan. Unwrap pork roast and place in roasting pan, atop aromatics (fat-side up).

5. Place in oven and roast for 30 minutes.

6. Reduce heat to 300°F and cook for an additional 30 minutes per pound, with a total cooking time of 4 hours and 30 minutes for an 8-pound roast.

7. Remove from oven and allow roast to rest, about 30 minutes.

8. Transfer to a cutting board and slice meat into 1/4 to 1/2-inch slices. Transfer slices to a platter and serve.

Sweet Desserts!

Sugar is a hard habit to break! Sweets are a decadent treat! And some people just got to have pie, cobbler or cake!

Oh, yeah, some folks do love cupcakes!

Me, I love cookies and Molasses Cookies are my favorite! Every time I see one it screams eat me!

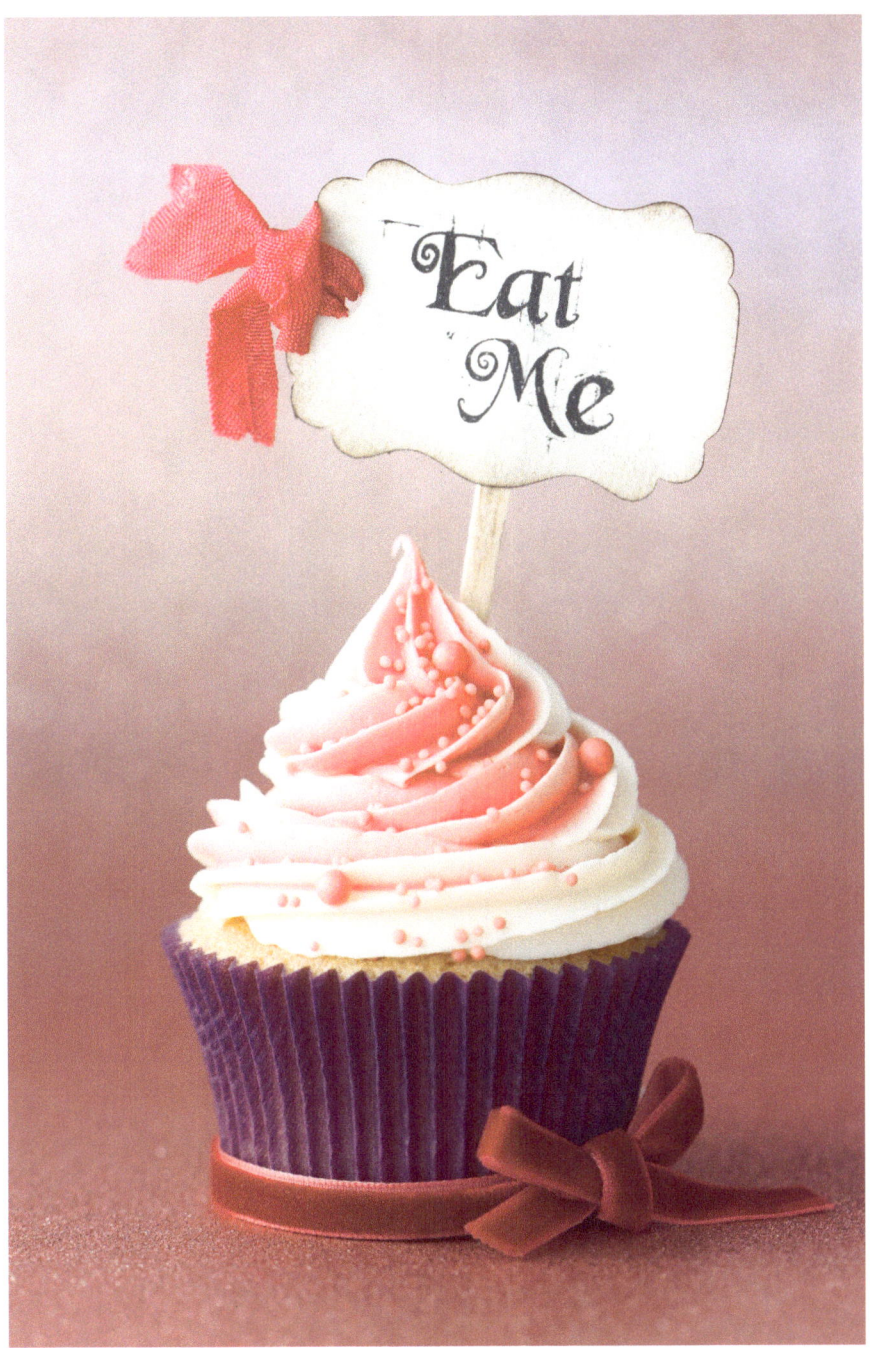

Soft Sweet Molasses Cookies!

Preheat oven to 375 degrees.

Ingredient:

- 1 1/2 cups butter, softened
- 1 cup granulated sugar
- 1 cup brown sugar
- 1/2 cup molasses
- 2 eggs
- 4 cups all-purpose flour
- 4 tsp. baking soda
- 2 tsp. ground cinnamon
- 1 tsp. ground cloves
- 1 tsp. ground ginger
- 1 1/2 tsp. Sea salt

Directions:

1. The most important thing to remember is to be sure to mix the wet Ingredients separately. Best practice to do is to mix the wet Ingredients together in a separate bowl and then the dry Ingredients together in a separate bowl. Combining them together later.
2. Preheat oven to 375 degrees.
3. Whisk together flour, soda, cinnamon, cloves, ginger and salt. Set aside.

SOFT SWEET MOLASSES COOKIES!

(These are your dry Ingredients.)

4. In a stand mixer (or with a handheld mixer), in a separate bowl, beat together butter and sugar on medium speed until light and fluffy, about 1-2 minutes. (These are your wet Ingredients.

5. Add in the eggs and molasses into the "WET" ingredients and beat on medium-low speed until combined.

6. Add in the dry Ingredients and beat together until combined.

7. Roll the dough into 1" diameter balls

8. Pour 1/4 cup of granulated sugar onto a shallow dish, and roll cookie balls in sugar to completely coat.

9. Place on cookie sheet at least 1 inch apart and bake for about 8-10 minutes.

10. Cookies will crack at the top, and the centers will still be a bit gooey.

11. Remove from oven and let cool for 2 minutes to firm slightly (if you move them too quickly off the baking sheet, they will fall apart), and then let cool completely or serve warm.

12. Cookies last up to one week in an airtight container (however in my home they never make it that long. (LOL).

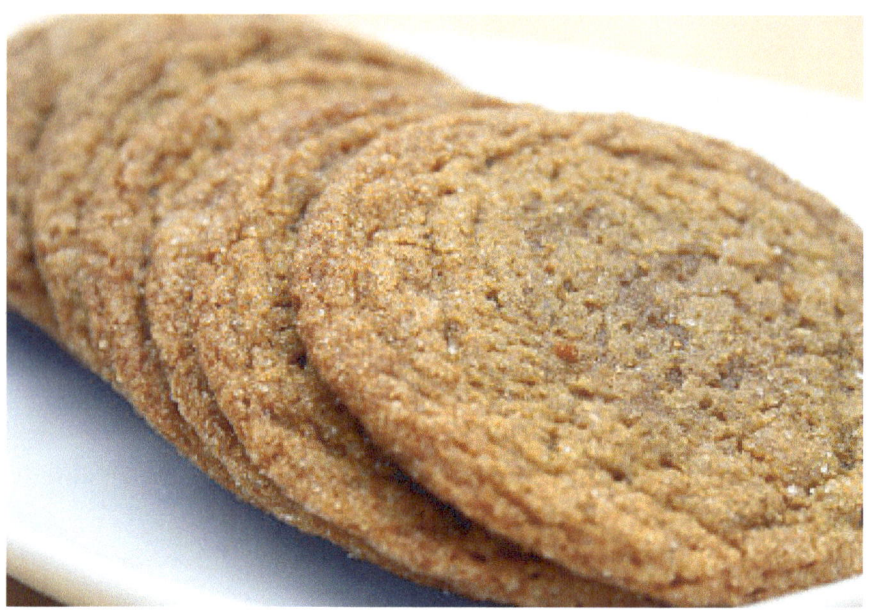

Chewy scrumptious Molasses Cookies!

Southern Tea Cookies Recipe!

Best kept secret to a perfect Tea Cookie is to make sure your Ingredients are room temperature...

Ingredients:

- 1 stick unsalted butter room temperature
- 3/4 cup granulated sugar
- 1 large egg at room temperature
- 2 teaspoons pure vanilla extract
- 1 1/2 cup all-purpose flour
- 1/4 teaspoon salt
- 1/4 teaspoon baking soda

Directions:

1. In a medium sized bowl, whisk together the flour, salt and baking soda and set aside.
2. In the bowl of your mixer, add butter and sugar and cream together on high speed until fluffy and smooth (about 4-5 minutes).
3. Turn mixer to medium speed and add in one egg and vanilla extract and beat until well incorporated.
4. Lastly, turn mixer to slow speed and add in flour mixture in intervals of three beating after each addition to incorporate.
5. After dough is well mixed, turn off mixer and remove dough from mixer

and add to a Ziploc bag and place in your refrigerator for at least one hour to firm up dough.

6. Once dough is firm, remove from fridge and preheat your oven to 325 degrees.

7. Line your cookie sheet with parchment paper.

8. Taking a measuring tablespoon, scoop out cookie dough the size of the tablespoon and roll into a ball. Using your thumb, gently press the center to flatten a bit and place on the tray.

9. Do the same for the rest of the dough leaving at least a 1 1/2 inches between each dough ball. **If you prefer you cookies cut into square shapes roll out dough on well greased cookie sheet and per-line into square shape before baking.

10. Bake for 9-11 minutes until golden brown on the edges and remove from the oven.

Cool for 5-10 minutes and serve.

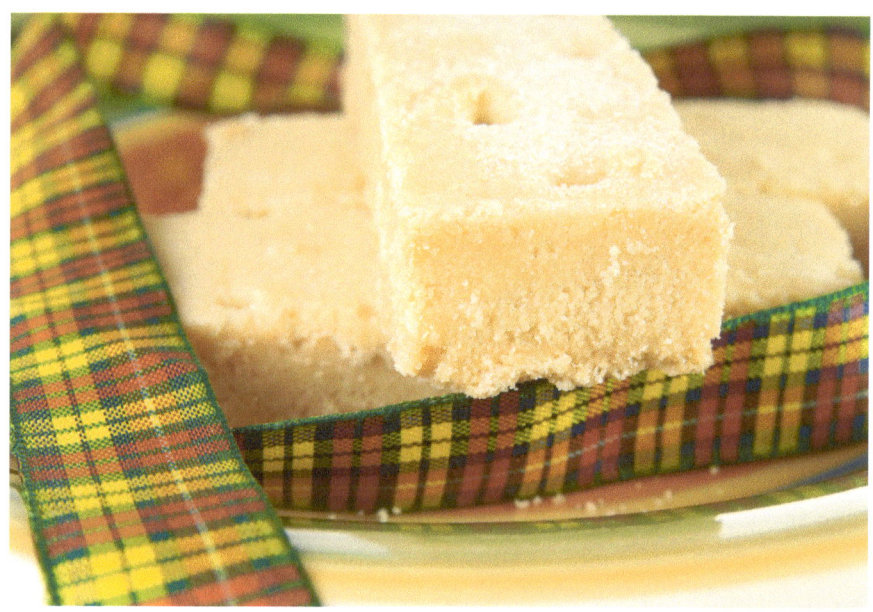

Old Fashioned Tea Cookies!

Homemade Moon Pies!

Ingredients:

The Vanilla Cookies

- 1/2 cup unsalted butter, softened
  - 1/2 cup granulated sugar
  - 1/4 cup packed light brown sugar
  - 1/2 teaspoon salt
  - 1 large egg
  - 1 egg yolk
  - 1 teaspoon vanilla extract
  - 1 3/4 cups all-purpose flour
  - 1 tablespoon cornstarch

FOR THE FILLING
  - 2 tablespoons water
  - 2 tablespoons light corn syrup
  - 1/3 cup granulated sugar
  - 1 egg white, room temperature
  - 1/2 tablespoon gelatin powder
  - 1 tablespoon cold water
  - 1/4 teaspoon vanilla extract

FOR THE CHOCOLATE GLAZE
  - 12 ounces semisweet chocolate, chopped

- 1 tablespoon vegetable oil

Directions:

How to Make the Vanilla Cookie Cookie for the Moon Pies

1. In a large mixing bowl, beat the butter, sugars, and salt together with an electric mixer on medium speed until well combined. Add the egg, egg yolk, and vanilla; beat until incorporated.

2. In a medium bowl, whisk the flour and cornstarch together. Add it to the butter mixture and beat until fully incorporated. Gather the dough into a ball, cover with plastic wrap and refrigerate for at least 2 hours.

3. Preheat the oven to 350°F. Scoop 1 tablespoon sized pieces of dough and roll them into balls. Place the balls of dough 2 inches apart on a baking sheet lined with parchment paper or silicon mat. Bake for 10 to 12 minutes or until the edges of the cookies are lightly browned.

4. Cool on the pan for 5 minutes, then transfer to a wire rack to cool completely.

MAKE THE FILLING

1. Combine the water, corn syrup, and sugar in a small saucepan fitted with a candy thermometer. Bring to a boil and cook to "soft-ball" stage, about 235°F.

2. Meanwhile, in a large bowl, beat the egg white on medium speed until soft peaks form.

3. Sprinkle the gelatin over the water and set aside to soften. Once the syrup reaches 235°F, add in the softened gelatin and mix until fully dissolved. With the mixer running on low, slowly pour the syrup into the beaten egg white. Add the vanilla. Turn the mixer to medium-high speed and continue to beat until stiff. (This may take around 3-5 minutes)

4. Transfer the marshmallow to a pastry bag fitted with a round tip. Pipe a large kiss of marshmallow on the bottom side of half the cookies. Top with a second cookie to form a sandwich. Refrigerate for 30 minutes.

MAKE THE GLAZE

1.Add chocolate and oil to a heatproof bowl and set it over a pot of barely simmering water. Stir constantly until chocolate is melted and smooth.

2.Working with one cookie at a time, use a fork to dip it into the bowl of melted chocolate. Flip it over to fully coat the cookie in chocolate. Tap off any excess and let it drop back into the bowl. Place the cookies on a wire rack set over a large baking sheet. Refrigerate until chocolate is set.

Keep cookies stored in the refrigerator until ready to serve. Cookies with keep for up to 3 days stored in an airtight container.

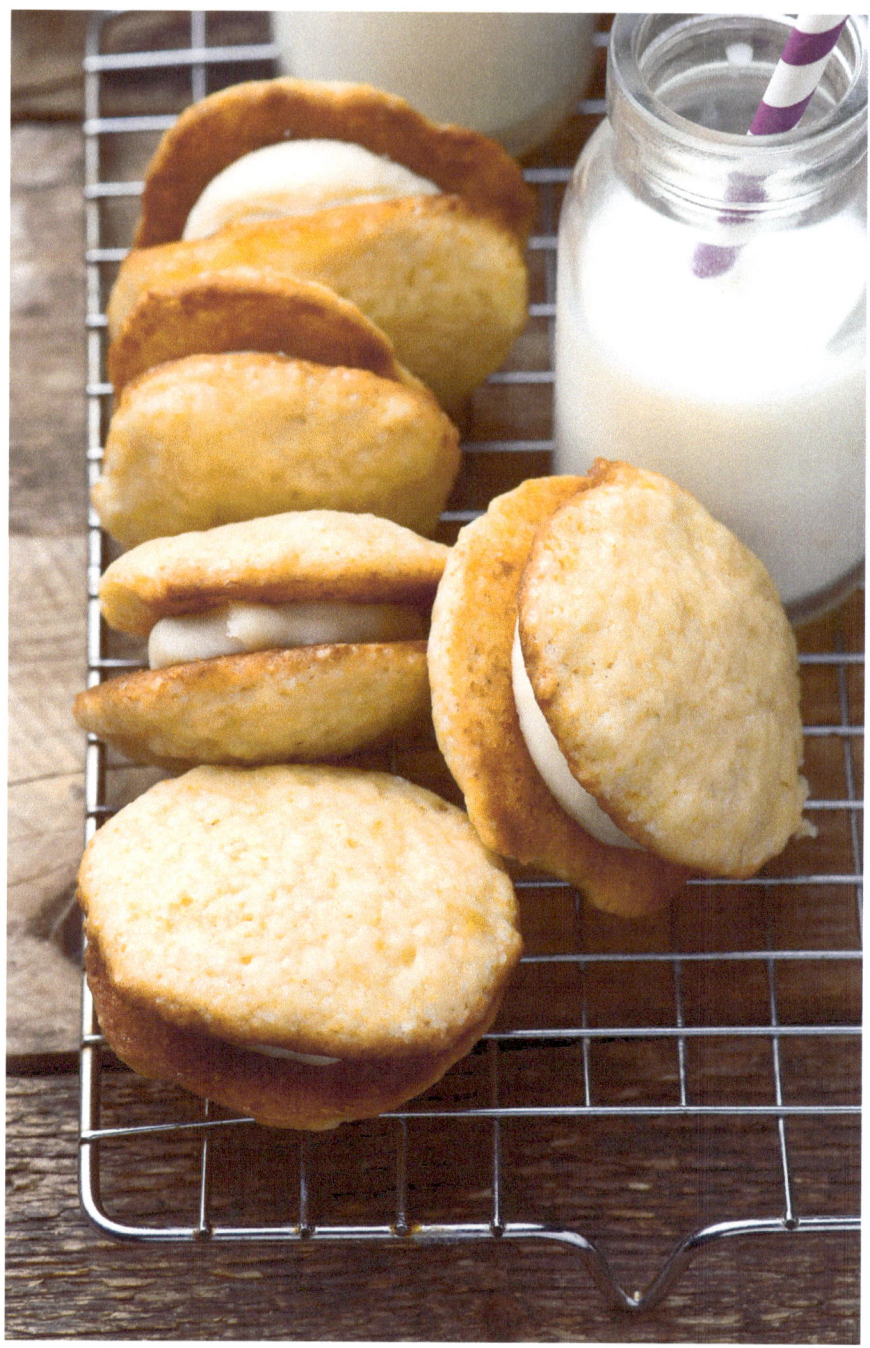

Moon Pie with a Chocolate Cookie!

Ingredients:

- 1/2 cup butter, softened
- 1 cup white sugar
- 1 egg
- 1 cup evaporated milk
- 1 teaspoon vanilla extract
- 2 cups all-purpose flour
- 1/2 teaspoon salt

How to Make the Chocolate Cookie

- 1/2 cup unsweetened cocoa powder
- 1 1/2 teaspoons baking soda
- 1/2 teaspoon baking powder
- 1/2 cup butter, softened
- 1 cup confectioners' sugar
- 1/2 teaspoon vanilla extract
- 1 cup marshmallow creme

Directions:

1. Preheat oven to 400 degrees F (200 degrees C). Lightly grease a cookie sheet.
2. To Make Cookie Crusts: In a large mixing bowl, cream together 1/2 cup butter or margarine and white sugar. Add egg, evaporated milk, and vanilla.

Mix well. In a separate bowl, mix together flour, salt, cocoa powder, baking soda, and baking powder. Add flour mixture slowly to sugar mixture while stirring. Mix just until all Ingredients are combined.

3.Drop the dough onto greased cookie sheet by rounded tablespoonfuls. Leave at least 3 inches in between each one; dough will spread as it bakes.

4.Bake in preheated oven for 6 to 8 minutes, until firm when pressed with finger. Allow to cool at least one hour before filling.

To Make Marshmallow Filling: In a medium mixing bowl, blend together 1/2 cup butter or margarine, confectioners' sugar, flavored extract, and marshmallow creme. Mix until smooth. Assemble pies by spreading 1 to 2 tablespoonfuls of filling on flat side of a cookie crust, then covering filling with flat side of another cookie crust.

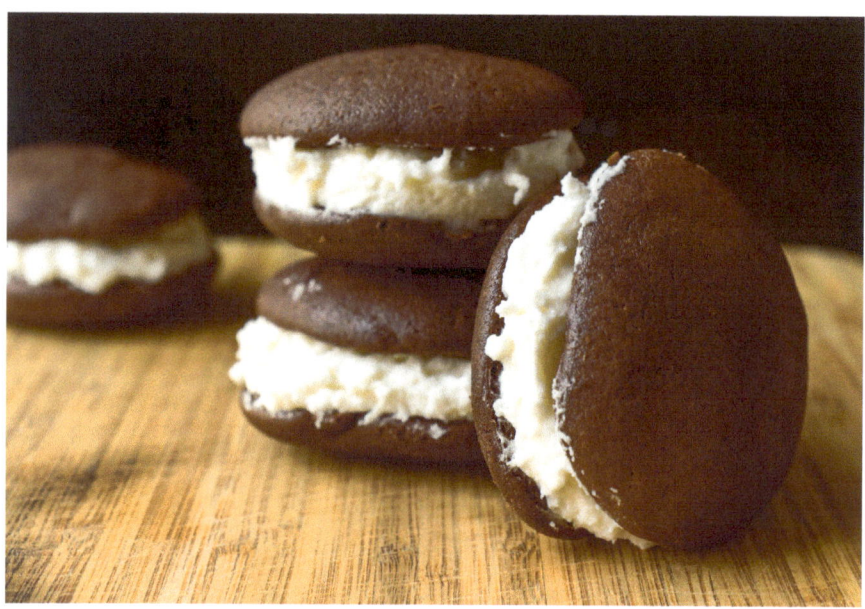

Chocolate Cookie Moon Pie!

Quick Semi Homemade Pie Crust Peach Cobbler!

Ingredients:

1 – 29 oz can sliced peaches in heavy syrup
   2/3 - cup sugar
   2 - tablespoons cornstarch
   2 - tablespoons. Butter
   ½ - teaspoon cinnamon
   1 teaspoon cinnamon & sugar mixed together for sprinkling on top
   2 - prepared roll-out ready-made pie crust.
   Preheat oven to 450*

Grease baking pan and line with one single pie crust. Drain peaches and reserve liquid.

Directions:

In a medium size pan mix sugar, cinnamon and cornstarch.

Stir in reserved peach juice/syrup (if you used canned peaches use the heavy syrup from the can.

Gradually bring to a boil. Boil 1-minute stirring constantly.

Add peaches and pour into a 1 ½ qt or 8 x 8 pasty lined baking dish.

Dot with butter sprinkle with sprinkle on cinnamon mixed with the sugar.

Top with second crust, brush with melted butter and sprinkle a little cinnamon sugar on top.

Bake 25-30 minutes.

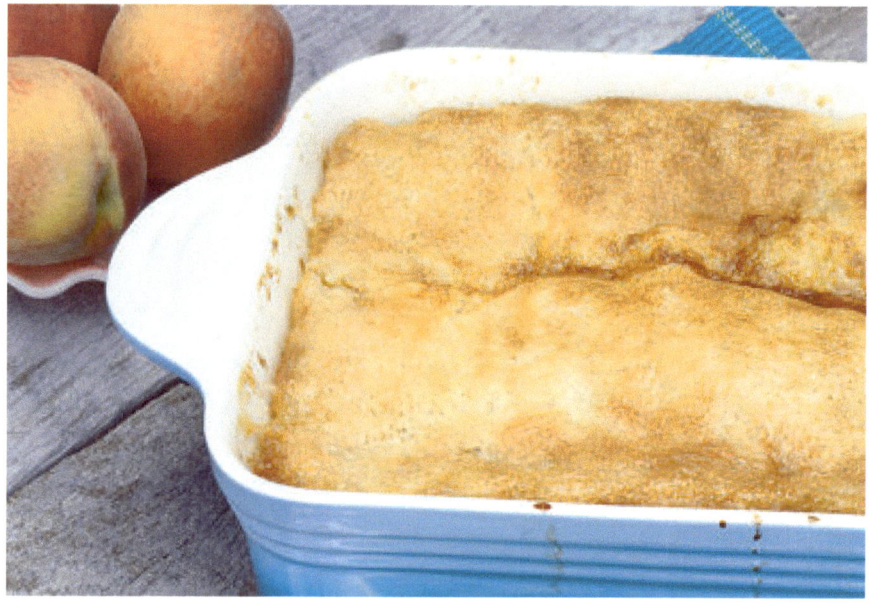

Peach Cobbler is always a favorite!

Quick Apple Pockets!

Ingredients:

·2 cup diced peeled apples
  ·1 tablespoon all-purpose flour
  ·1/2 1/1/2 teaspoon ground cinnamon
  ·1/2 cup butter, softened
  ·1 cup sugar
  ·2 tablespoons of coarse Sugar – Also known as pearl or decorating sugar or crystal sugar. Sprinkle on top before baking for decorations. *optional
  ·1/2 teaspoon vanilla extract
  ·1 box ready-made roll out pie crust (can use puff pastry also)

Directions:

Heat oven to 400° F. Unroll pie crusts on work surface. Cut each crust into quarters, making 8 wedges.

Mix apples, sugar, flour and cinnamon. Top half of each crust wedge with 1/3 cup apple mixture. Fold sides of wedges over filling. With fork, press edges to seal. Place on ungreased cookie sheet. Cut several small slits in top of each to allow steam to escape. Sprinkle with coarse/crystal sugar *optional

*(Optional if you use puff pastry be sure to seal edges. Fold over from corner to corner into a triangle shape, and press edges together to seal.)

Bake 15 to 20 minutes or until light golden brown. Serve warm or cool.

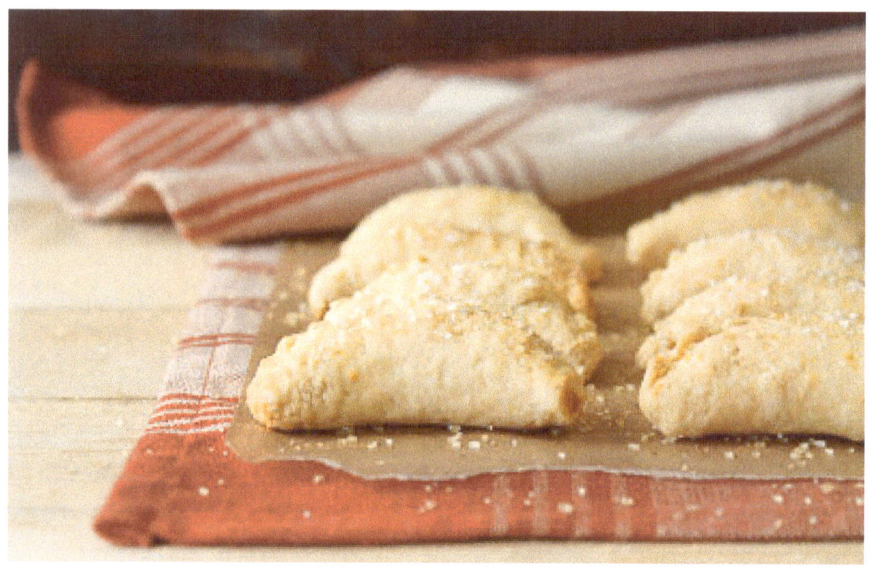

Quick Apple Pockets! Some call Apple Hand Pies!

Old Fashion Homemade Pecan Squares!

Ingredients:

- 2 cups all-purpose flour
  - 2/3 cup powdered sugar
  - 2/3 cup butter
  - 1/2 cup packed light brown sugar
  - 1/2 cup honey
  - 3 tablespoons whipping cream
  - 1 3 ½ cups coarsely chopped pecans *(Walnuts also work well with this recipe)*

Directions:

Sift together 2 cups flour and 2/3 cup powdered sugar. Cut in 3/4 cup softened butter using a pastry blender or fork just until mixture resembles coarse meal. Pat mixture on bottom and 1 1/2 inches up sides of a lightly greased 13- x 9-inch baking dish.

Step 1
Bake at 350° for 20 minutes or until edges are lightly browned. Cool.

Step 2
Bring brown sugar, honey, 2/3 cup butter, and whipping cream to a boil in a saucepan over medium-high heat. Stir in pecans and pour hot filling into prepared crust.

Step 3

Bake at 350° for 25 to 30 minutes or until golden and bubbly. Cool completely before cutting into 2-inch squares.

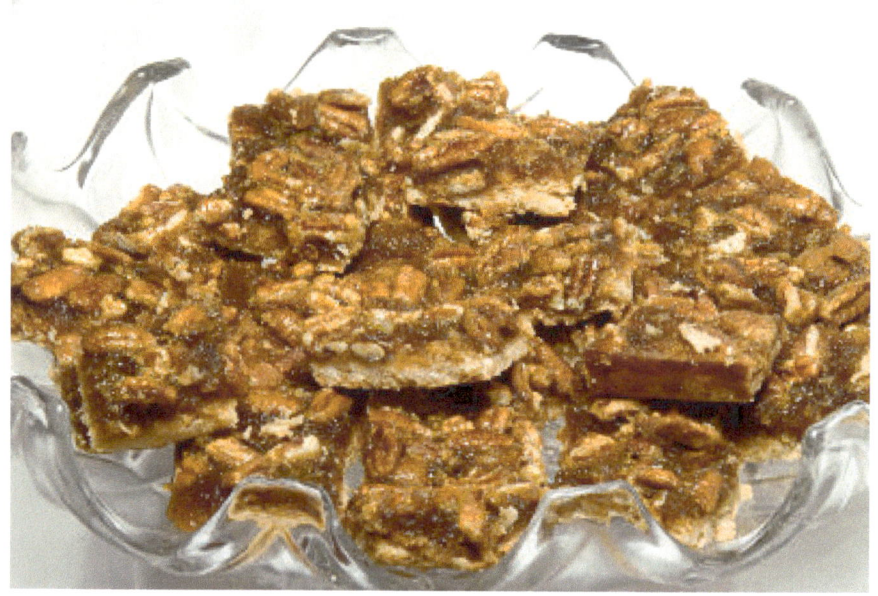

Semi Home-Made Quick Pecan Squares!

Ingredients:

- 2 cups all-purpose flour
  - 1/2 cup confectioners' sugar
  - 1 cup butter, softened
  - 1 can (14 ounces) sweetened condensed milk
  - 1 large egg, room temperature
  - 1 teaspoon vanilla extract
  - Pinch salt
  - 1 package (8 ounces) milk chocolate English toffee bits
  - 1 cup chopped pecans
  - **Sheet of clear plastic wrap**

Directions:

- In a large bowl, combine flour and sugar. Cut in butter until mixture resembles coarse meal. Next pour flour batter into a 13 x 9 greased baking dish. Place the clear plastic wrap on top of flour dough and press firmly onto the bottom of a greased 13 x 9-in. baking dish (remove the clear plastic wrap before placing into the oven). Bake at 350° for 15 minutes.
  - Meanwhile, in large bowl, beat the milk, egg, vanilla and salt until smooth. Stir in toffee bits and pecans; spread evenly over baked crust.
  - Bake until lightly browned, 20-25 minutes longer. Cool. Cover and chill;

cut into bars. Store in refrigerator.

*For an added flavor: Do you love toffee and caramel or toffee and chocolate? Then try this optional favor enhancer.

**Optional – can add 1/2 bag of either caramel baking chips or chocolate baking chips to the wet mixture before pouring into the baked pie crust. Try it you might love it!

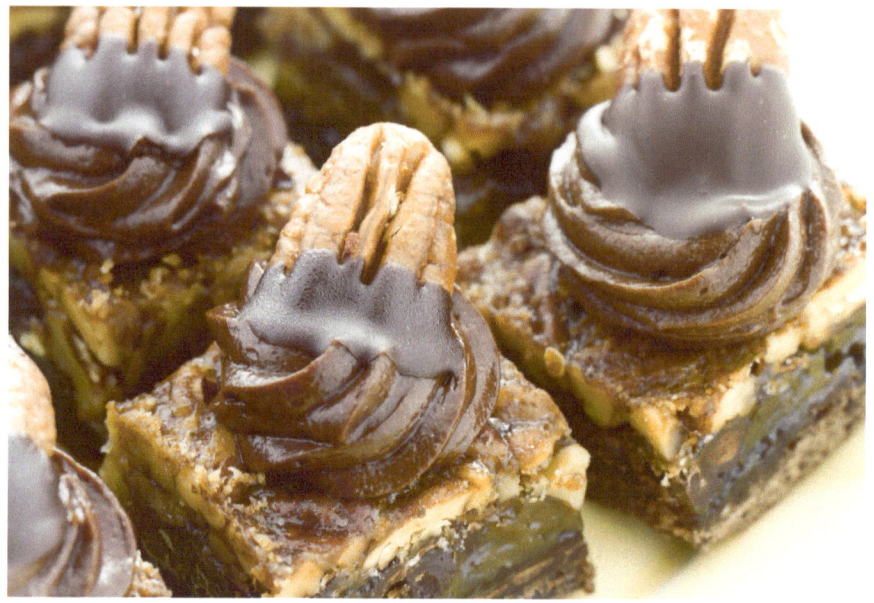

Enhance your Pecan Square with Chocolate or Caramel!

Homemade Old-Fashioned Lost Pies of the South!

The Black Apple is native to Benton County, Arkansas. It originated in the mid-19th Century in Benton Arkansas. These tree growing apples are normally medium in size with a flattened shape and is said to be a firm, tart and juicy fruit.

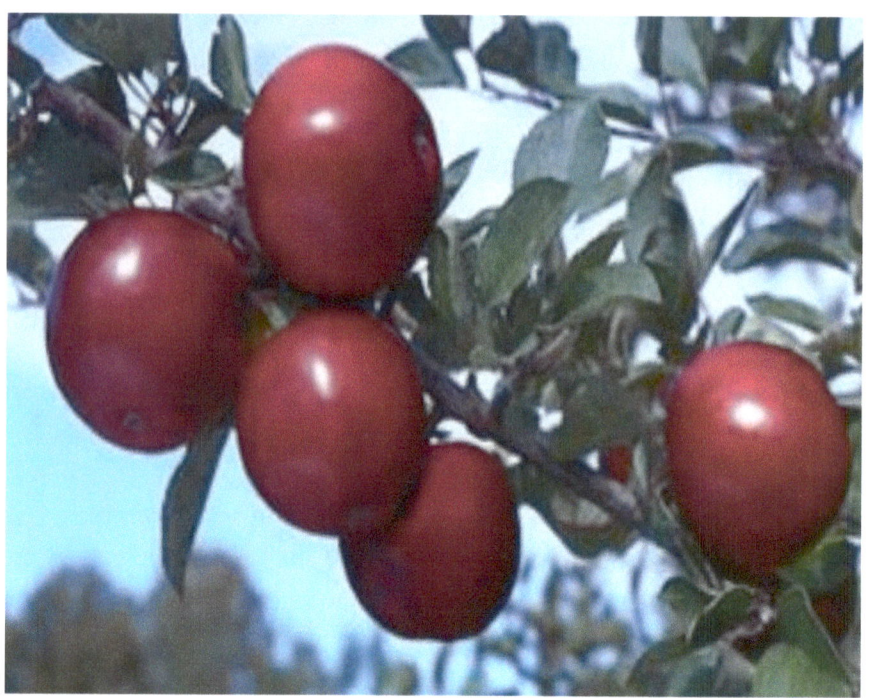

The Black Apple!

Arkansas Black Apple Pie!

Arkansas Black Apple Pie Filling

Preheat oven to 425°F.

Ingredients:

·5 to 6 Arkansas Black or Granny Smith apples (about 3 1/2 lb.), peeled and thinly sliced

- ·1 tablespoon fresh lemon juice (from 1 lemon) or apple cider vinegar
- ·1 cup granulated sugar
- ·1/4 cup all-purpose flour
- ·1 teaspoon ground cinnamon
- ·1/2 teaspoon freshly grated or ground nutmeg
- ·1/4 teaspoon ground allspice
- ·1/4 teaspoon kosher salt

Directions:

Turn down oven to *oven to 350°F bake pie crust for ten minutes before adding filling.*

    Prepare the Apple Filling: Place apples and fresh lemon juice in a large bowl; toss well to coat. Stir together granulated sugar, flour, ground cinnamon, freshly grated nutmeg, ground allspice, and kosher salt in a bowl; add to apple mixture and toss well to combine.

Next pour the filling into the pie crust. Loosely cover pie with aluminum foil. Bake at 350°F until crust is golden brown, apples are tender, and juices are bubbly, 1 hour to 1 hour and 10 minutes.

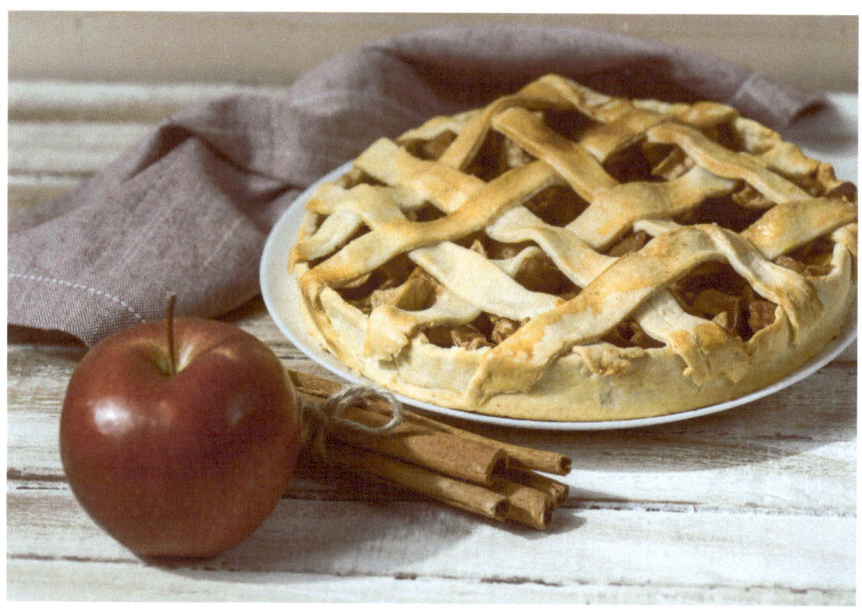

Arkansas Black Apple Pie!

Old Time Pie Crust Made With Vinegar!

Pie Crust Ingredients:

- 2 teaspoons distilled white vinegar
- 5 tablespoons ice water
- 1-1/4 cup Crisco (vegetable Shortening)
- 3 cups All-purpose Flour
- 1 whole Egg
- 5 Tablespoons Cold Water
- 1 Tablespoon White Vinegar
- 1 teaspoon Salt

Directions:

1. In a large bowl, mix flour and salt. With a pastry blender, cut in the shortening until it resembles pea-sized, this takes about 4 minutes with a pastry cutter, little longer if using a folk.

2. Beat together egg, vinegar and water. Mix liquid with flour mixture, using a fork, until mixture forms a ball (Note: add liquid one tablespoon at a time. You probably will not use all of it.)

3. Roll out on lightly floured pastry cloth with cloth covered roller.

4. Brush the crust with milk and sprinkle with sugar before baking.

THE SWEET PEPPER CAJUN! TASTY SOULFUL FOOD COOKBOOK!

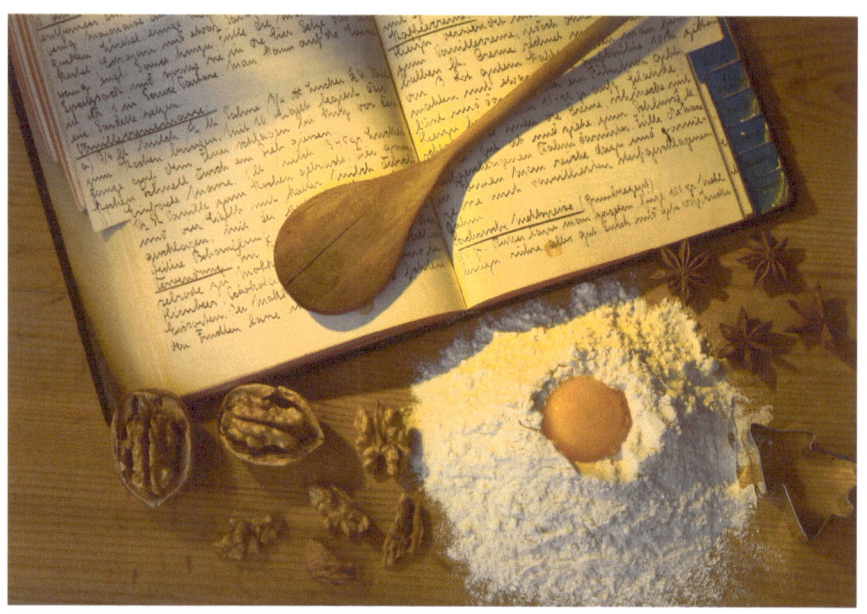

Lost Stacked Sweet Potato Pie Recipe!

Preheat oven to 350°F

Sweet Potato Filling

- 3 pounds sweet potatoes (about 6 medium-size sweet potatoes, cut each slice about 2 inches in diameter round- should resemble round disk)
  - 1 1/4 cups granulated sugar
  - 2 tablespoons all-purpose flour
  - 1/4 teaspoon ground allspice
  - 1/2 teaspoon ground ginger
  - 1/2 teaspoon ground nutmeg
  - 1/4 teaspoon ground cloves
  - 1/4 cup sorghum syrup or molasses or pure cane syrup or honey
  - 1/3 cup cold unsalted butter, chopped into small pieces
- EGG WASH
  - 1 large egg
  - 1 tablespoon water
  - 2 tablespoons granulated sugar (optional)

Directions:

1.Prepare the Crust: Unwrap chilled pie dough disks from Double-Crust Pie Pastry, and place on a lightly floured surface. Let stand at room temperature until slightly softened, about 5 minutes. Sprinkle each disk with flour. Roll 1 disk into a 12-inch circle. Carefully fit dough circle into a 9-inch deep-dish glass pie plate, leaving a 1 1/2-inch overhang. Refrigerate until ready to use. Roll remaining disk into a 10-inch circle, and refrigerate until ready to use.

2. Prepare the Sweet Potato Filling: Place whole, unpeeled sweet potatoes in a large pot with water to cover by 2 inches. Bring to a rolling boil over high. Reduce heat to medium, maintaining a gentle boil. Cook until sweet potatoes are just tender enough to be sliced, but not so tender that they fall apart, 25 to 35 minutes. (Remove any smaller sweet potatoes as they are done, allowing larger ones to cook until they reach the ideal texture.)

3. Stir together sugar, flour, allspice, ginger, nutmeg, and cloves in a small bowl.

4. Drain sweet potatoes, and transfer to a platter to cool. Peel potatoes; trim and discard any fibers. Cut potatoes crosswise into 1/4-inch-thick rounds. (You will need about 4 cups to generously fill piecrust.) Gently toss sweet potatoes with sugar-spice mixture.

5. Preheat oven to 350°F. Cover bottom of piecrust in pie plate with a layer of Sweet Potato Filling; continue to layer to fill piecrust. Add additional filling to center, building it up a little higher than outer edges. Sprinkle all remaining sugar-spice mixture in bowl over top of pie; drizzle with sorghum syrup, and dot with butter pieces.

6. Carefully place 10-inch dough circle over filling. Fold edges of bottom crust up and over edges of top crust, and press firmly to seal. Using the tines of a fork, press dough around piecrust edge to make a decorative design. Using a sharp knife, cut 8 slits in top piecrust for steam to escape.

7. Prepare the Egg Wash: Stir together egg and water in a small bowl. Using a pastry brush, brush egg mixture evenly over piecrust. Sprinkle sugar over crust, if desired. Place pie on a baking sheet.

8. Bake in preheated oven until crust is browned, filling is bubbly, and sweet potatoes are tender all the way through, about 1 hour.

LOST STACKED SWEET POTATO PIE RECIPE!

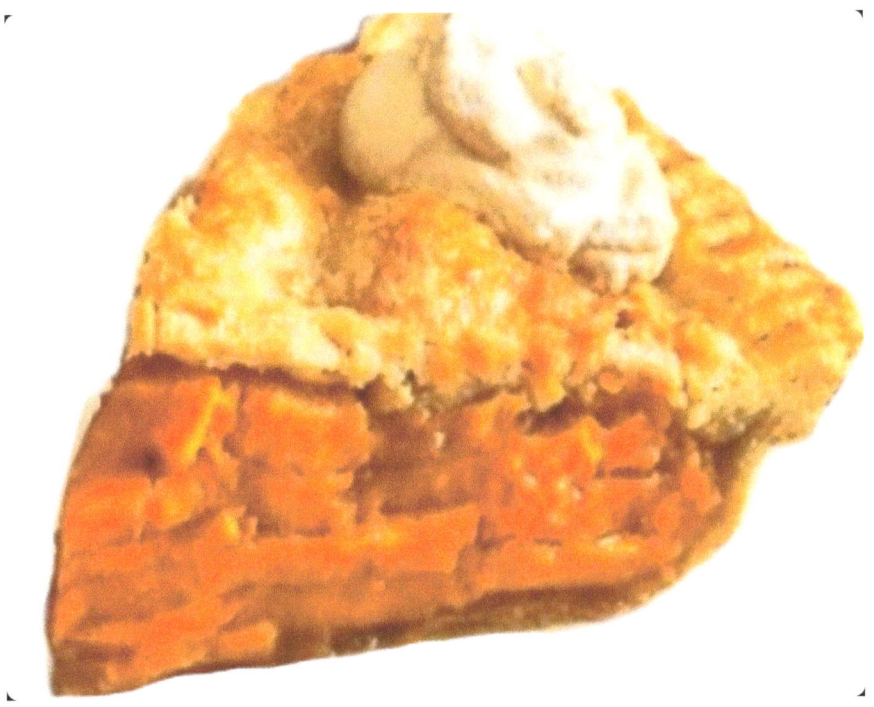

Old Fashion Stacked Sweet Potato Pie!

Slap Ya Mamma Cajun Meat Pies!

Ingredients:

- 1½ pounds ground beef
- 1½ pounds ground pork
- 1 cup chopped onions
- 1 cup chopped green pepper
- 2 tablespoons minced parsley
- 2 tablespoons garlic puree
- 1 tablespoon Slap Ya Mamma Cajun Seasoning
- 1 teaspoon black pepper
- 1 teaspoon red pepper
- ½ cup bread crumbs
- 2 cups self-rising flour, sifted
- ⅓ cup shortening
- ¾ cup milk
- 1 egg, beaten
- 1 teaspoon of distilled white vinegar

Directions:

Cook meat, chopped up vegetables and seasoning over medium heat until meat is brown. Stir breadcrumbs over meat mixture. Remove from heat and let cool slightly. Drain mixture in a strainer or colander and set aside.

Make the Dough

Sift flour into a medium bowl. Cut in shortening until mixture resembles coarse crumbs. Add 1 teaspoon of distilled white vinegar, milk and egg. Stir with a fork until ingredients are moistened. Shape dough into a ball and divide into 3 balls.

Working 1 at a time, roll each dough ball out on a floured surface to 1/8-inch thickness; cut into 5½-inch circles using a saucer as a guide.

Transfer to a lightly greased baking sheet and divide meat mixture evenly on one side of each dough circle. Moisten edges with a bit of water and fold pastry over to cover filling. Seal edges using a fork dipped in water. Prick pastry gently with a fork. Working in batches, deep fry in hot oil (350 F) until golden brown. Drain on paper towels and serve warm.

**Can use box ready-made roll out pie crust or puff pastry.

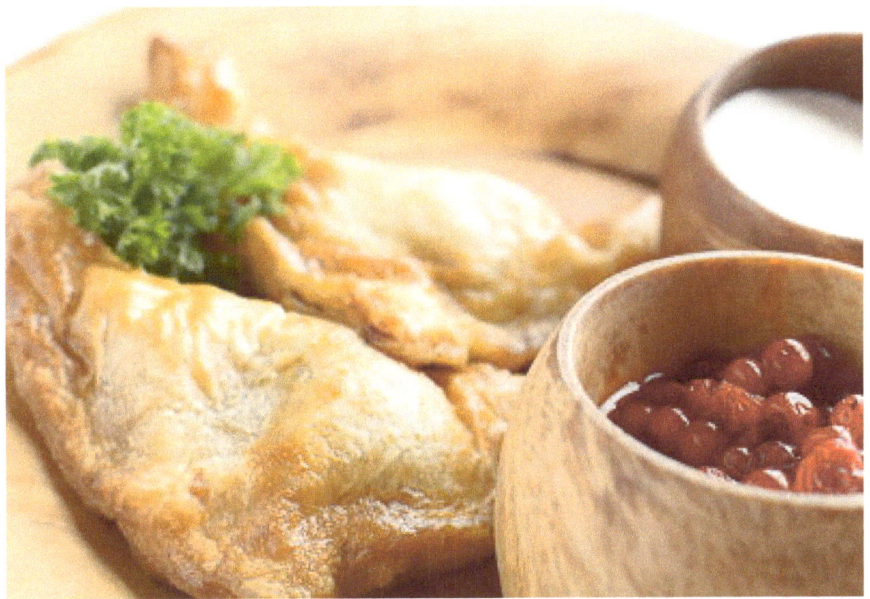

Meat Pies Made with Puff Pastry!

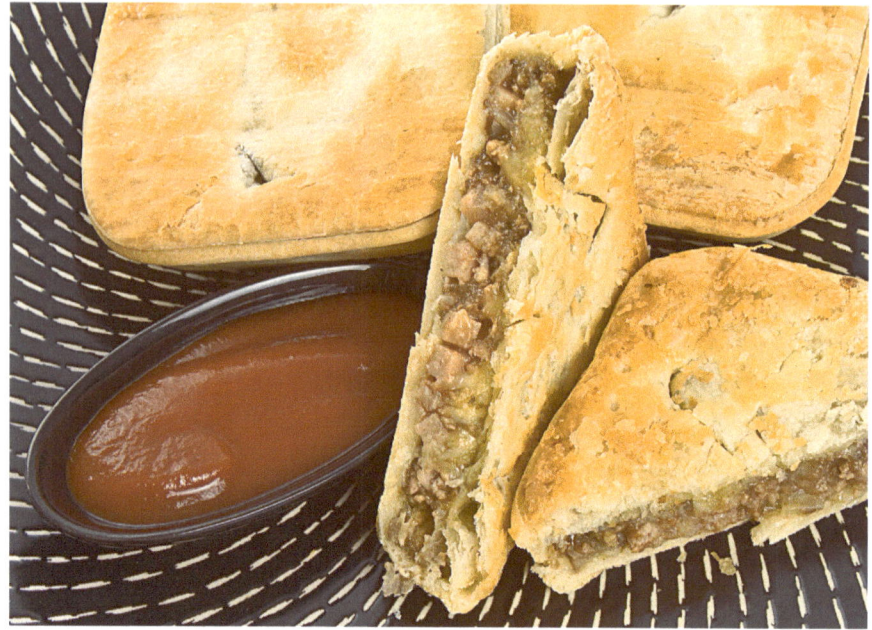

Meat Pies Made with Pie Crust!

* * *

Old Time Pie Crust Made With Vinegar

Pie Crust Ingredients:

·2 teaspoons distilled white vinegar
- ·5 tablespoons ice water
- ·1-1/4 cup Crisco (vegetable Shortening)
- ·3 cups All-purpose Flour
- ·1 whole Egg
- ·5 Tablespoons Cold Water
- ·1 Tablespoon White Vinegar

·1 teaspoon Salt

Directions:

1.In a large bowl, mix flour and salt. With a pastry blender, cut in the shortening until it resembles pea-sized, this takes about 4 minutes with a pastry cutter, little longer if using a folk.

2. Beat together egg, vinegar and water. Mix liquid with flour mixture, using a fork, until mixture forms a ball (Note: add liquid one tablespoon at a time. You probably will not use all of it.)

3. Roll out on lightly floured pastry cloth with cloth covered roller.

4.Brush the crust with milk and sprinkle with sugar before baking.

Beverages/Drinks/Punches/Smoothies!

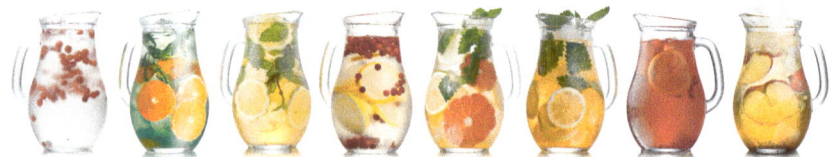

Drinks- Punches- Smoothies!

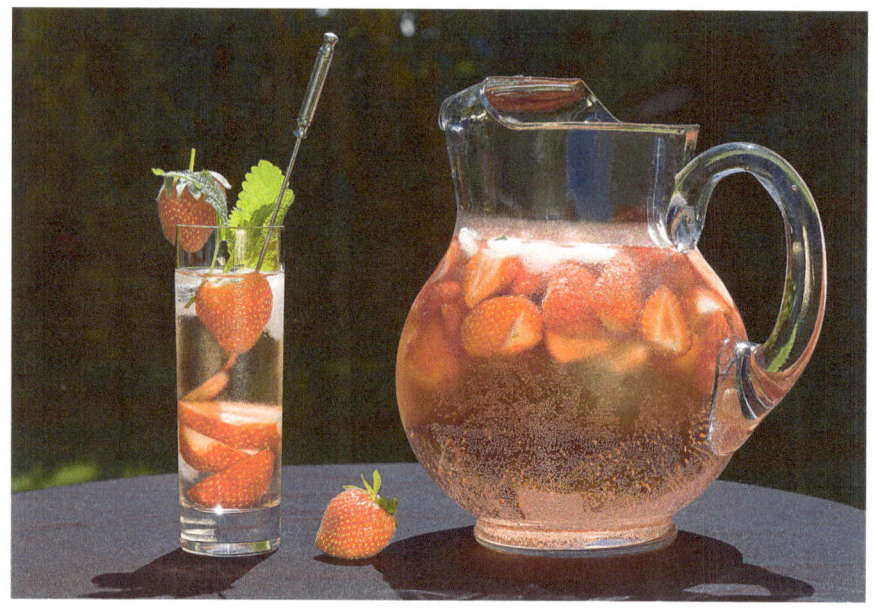

Mock Strawberry Champagne Punch!

BEVERAGES/DRINKS/PUNCHES/SMOOTHIES!

Tasty Watermelon Punch!

Ingredients:

- **2 cup** watermelon Cubs (deseeded)
- **1-inch fresh** ginger (peeled)
- **2 tbsp** sugar
- **1/2 cup** pineapple
- **1 tbsp** lemon juice
- **to taste** Salt
- **1 glass** sparkling water
- Few ice cubes and watermelon for garnishing

Directions:

- Take a mixture jar.
- Add watermelon, pineapple, sugar, lemon juice, ginger and salt.
- Grind it well.
- Add little water if require.
- Stir the mixture. (Optional)
- Now in a serving glass add the mixture.
- Pour sparkling water.
- Mix it well.
- Serve with watermelon and ice cubes.

TASTY WATERMELON PUNCH!

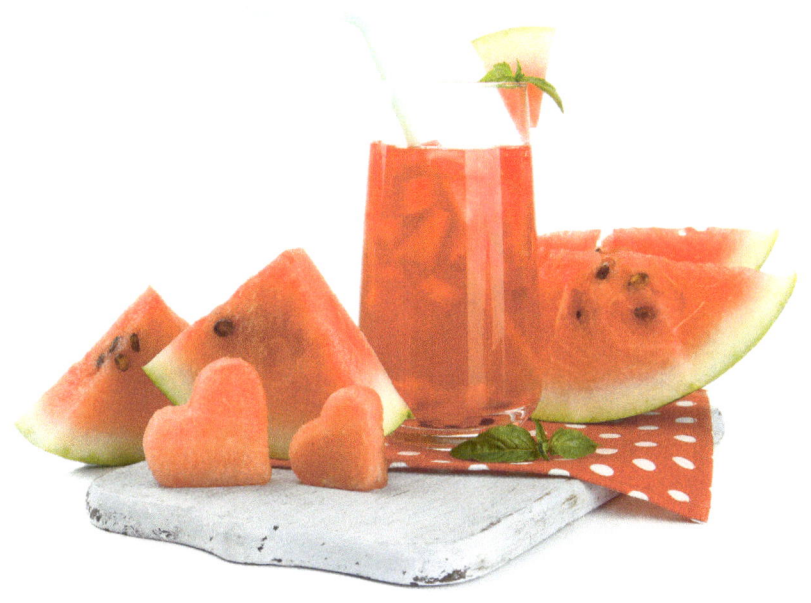

Fruity Homemade Punch!

Ingredients:

- 3 slices pineapple
- 1 tablespoon lime juice
- 1/2 cup grapefruit
- 1/2 orange juice
- 3 oranges
- 1 small apple
- 1/2 cup green grapes
- 1 kiwi sliced
- 1/2 cup cherries
- 1/4 cup pomegranate
- 5-6 scooped outs of watermelon
- 3/4 cup ginger ale
- 6 ice cubes
- 1 Lemon slice to garnish
- 2 sprigs mint

Directions:

- Take out the fresh juice of oranges, pineapple and grapefruit.
- Strain it in a pitcher and add lemon juice, Add crushed ice to it
- By then chop apple, grapes and slice kiwi too, Take out the kernels of

pomegranate, Scoop watermelon too
- Now just before serving, add ginger ale to the juice pitcher
- Add some more crushed ice in the glasses.
- Add fruit pieces. Pour juice over it.
- Garnish with mint leaves and serve chilled.

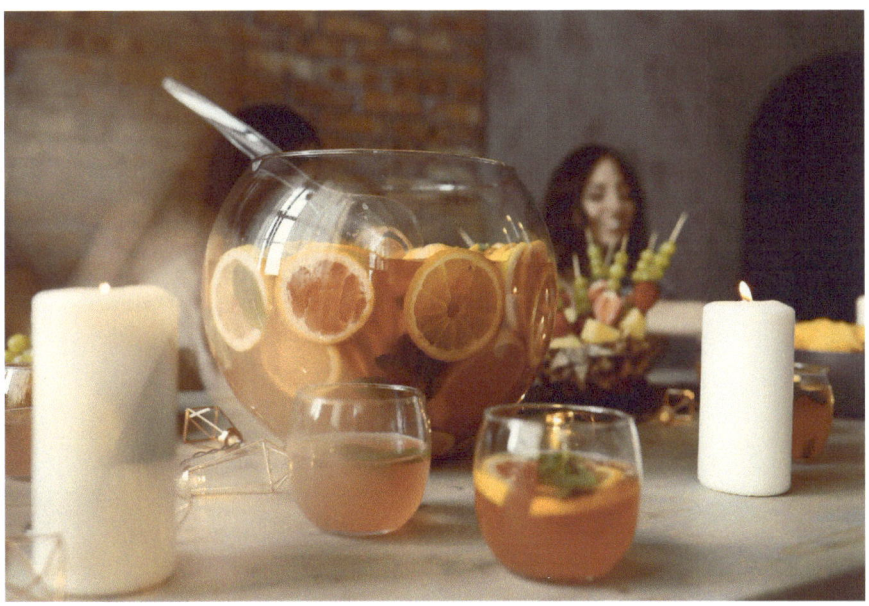

Fruit Punch is always quenches a crowd's thirst!

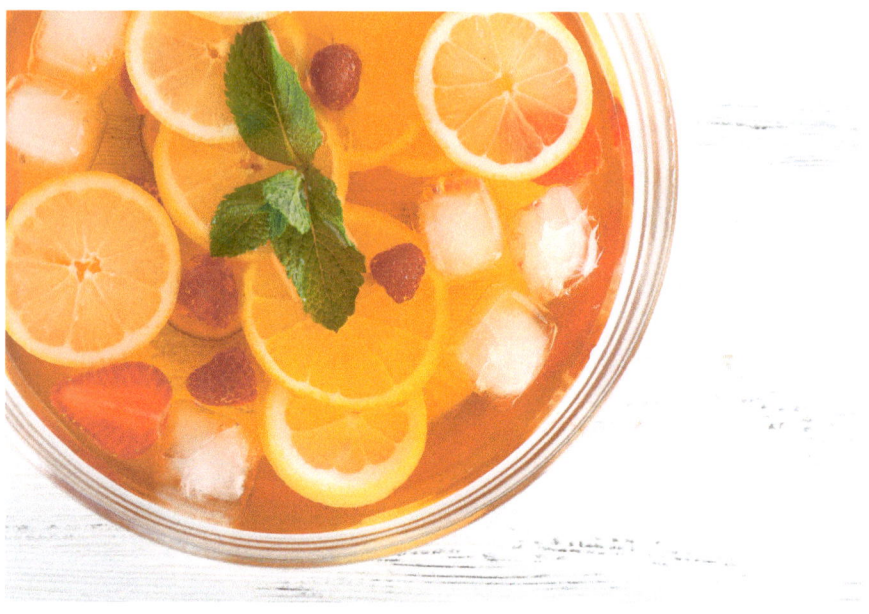

Mock Champagne Punch!

Mock Champagne Punch

Ingredients:

·1-quart white grape juice, chilled
 ·1-quart ginger ale, chilled
 ·Strawberries or raspberries *optional banana slices*

Directions:

·Combine grape juice and ginger ale; pour into a punch bowl or glasses. Garnish with berries.

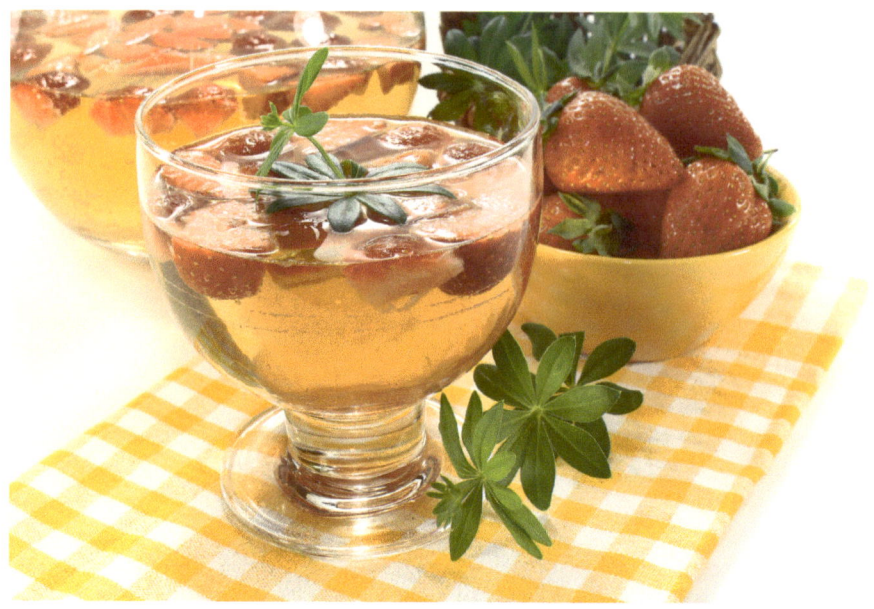

Mock Champagne Punch With Berries!

MOCK CHAMPAGNE PUNCH!

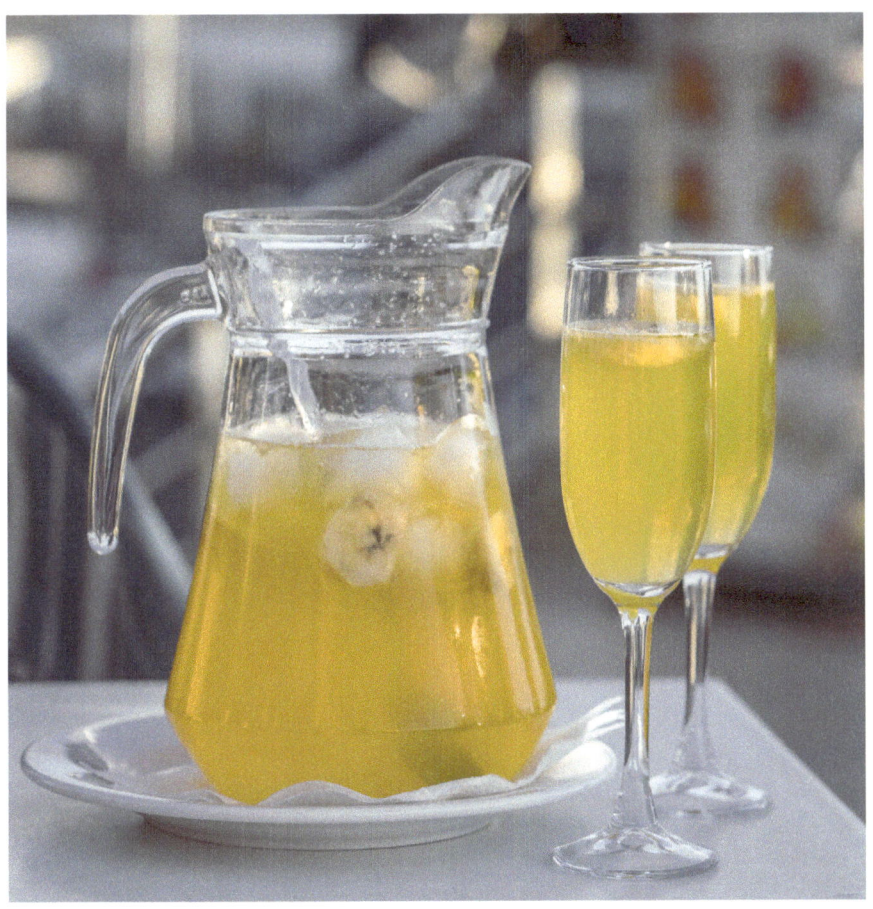

Mock Champagne Punch With Bananas Slices!

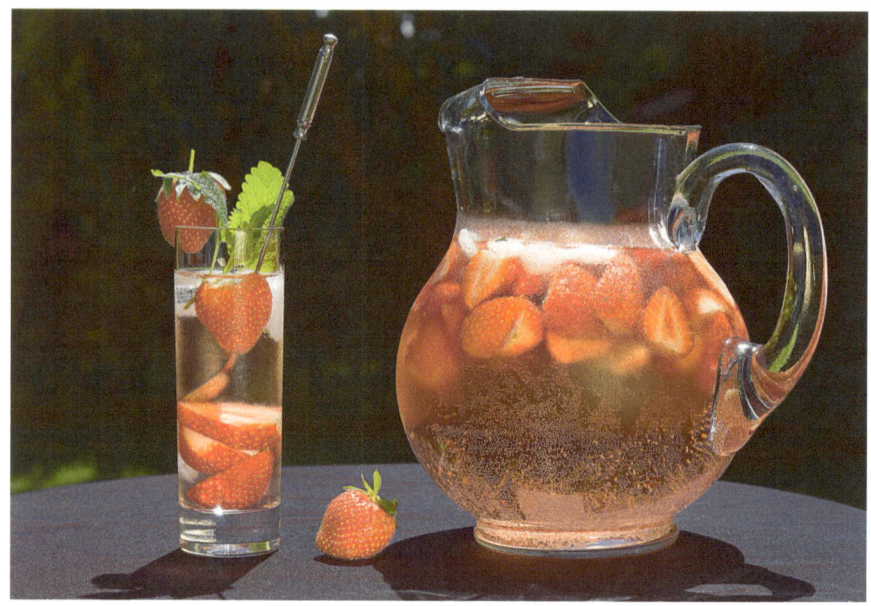

Mock Strawberry Champagne Punch!

Ingredients:

- 1-quart Jumex Strawberry Nectar from concentrated, chilled
- 1-quart ginger ale, chilled
- Strawberries

Directions:

- Combine Jumex Strawberry Nectar and ginger ale; pour into a punch bowl or glasses. Garnish with strawberries.

Fruity Berry Smoothie!

Ingredients:

- 1 cup banana
  - 1 cup frozen strawberries
  - 1 cup frozen blackberries, plus more for garnish (optional)
  - 1 cup frozen raspberries
  - 1 1/4 cup almond milk
  - 1/2 cup Greek yogurt

Directions:

1. In a blender, combine all Ingredients and blend until smooth.
2. Divide between 2 cups and top with blackberries, if desired.

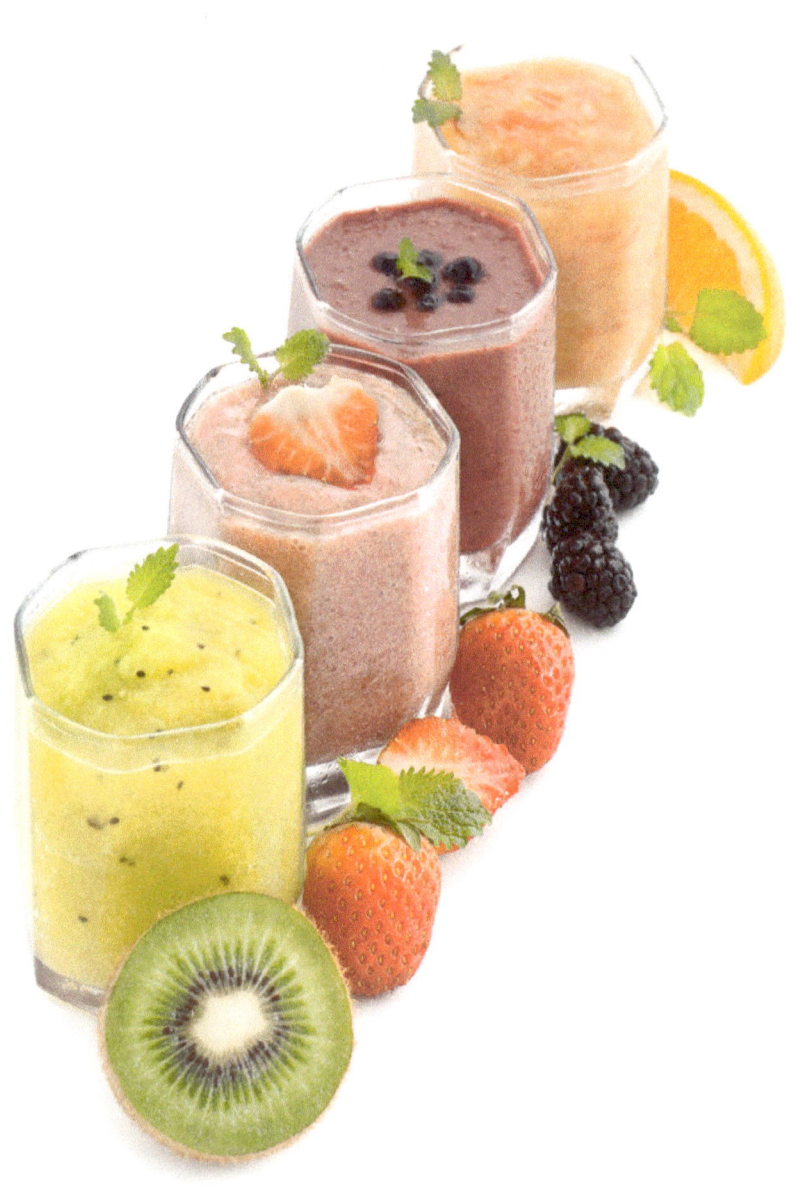

Make your smoothie your very own!

FRUITY BERRY SMOOTHIE!

Homemade Iced Tea!

Ingredients:

Lipton Tea or your favorite brand
·Lime
·Water
·Optional sugar syrup to taste. (Sugar syrup is one-part granulated sugar and one-part water bring to a boil and then allowed to cool. Use to flavor any beverages you should desire.)
·For One Gallon Size – 6 to 8 tea bags per gallon and sugar to taste.

Directions:

Lipton, hot water and sugar were placed in a jug. After simmering a dash of lime was squeezed. Lime wages were cut and added. Chilled ice water was added and served.

HOMEMADE ICED TEA!

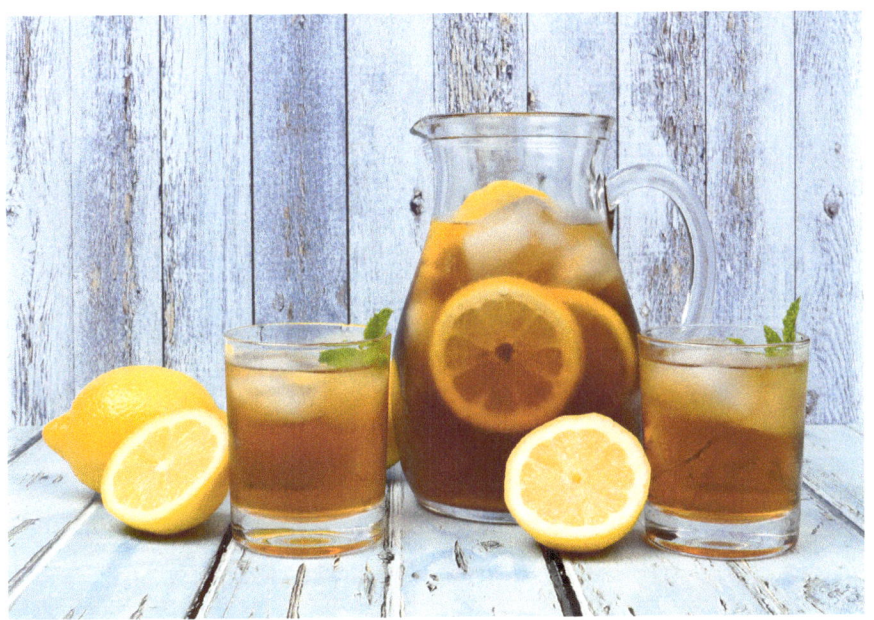

Holidays & Special Occasions!

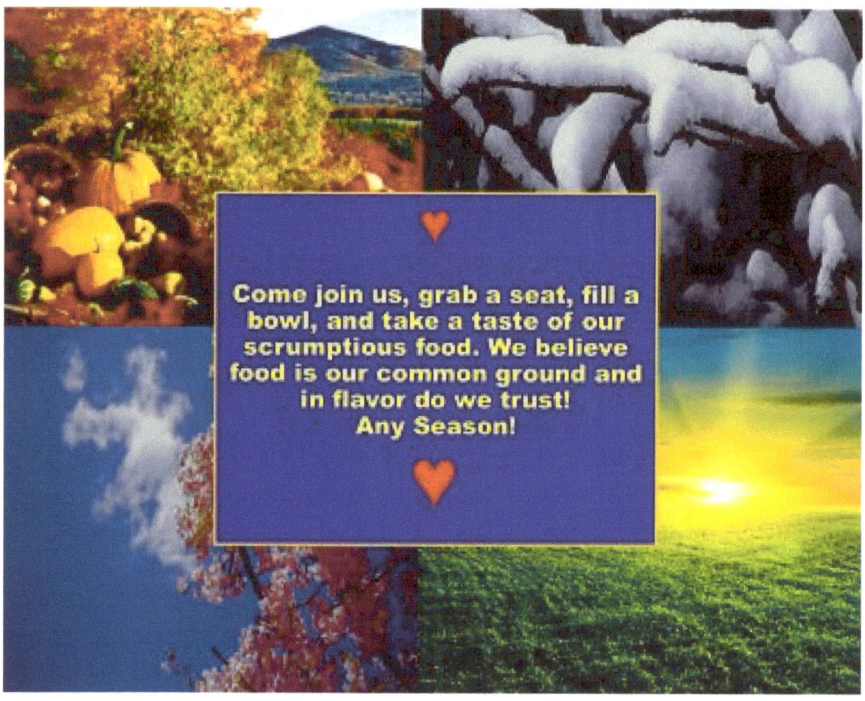

Holidays & Special Occasions Menus!

**Enjoy These Menus for Thanksgiving Feast, Christmas Feast or New Year's!
They All Aim To Please A Large Crowd!**

HOLIDAYS & SPECIAL OCCASIONS!

Menu
Southern Cornbread Dressing
Creole Roasted Turkey
Sweet Candied Sweet Potatoes
Hickory Smoked Collard Greens
Angel Biscuits

Menu
Pineapple Brown Sugar Glazed Ham
Creamy Cheesy Scalloped Potatoes
Roasted Holiday Veggies
Butternut Squash & Andouille Dressing
Cranberry Salad Mold
Mamma's Million Dollar Pound Cake
30 Minute Dinner Rolls

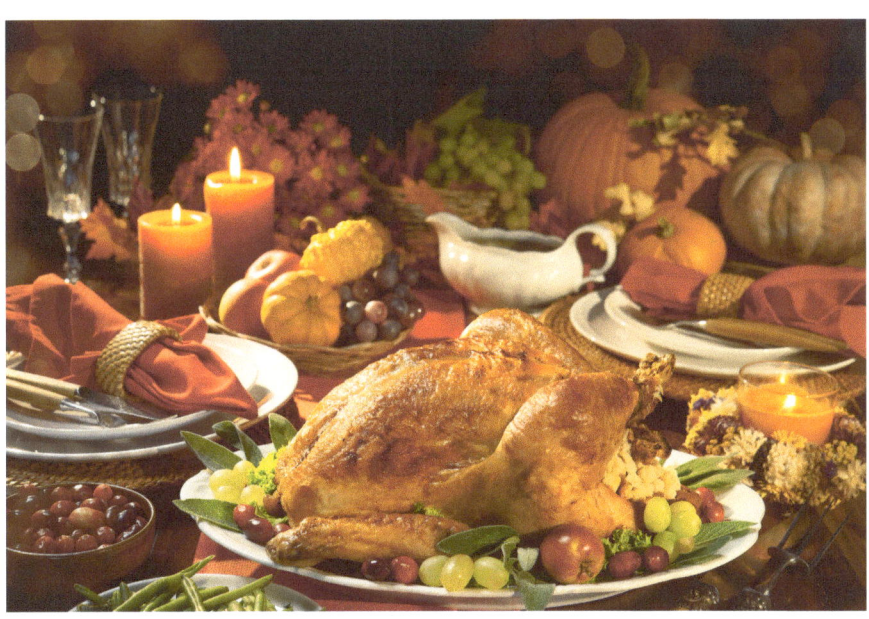

Southern Cornbread Dressing!

Note: The cornbread should be made ahead.

Ingredients:

Cornbread
- 1 cup self-rising cornmeal
- 1/2 cup self-rising flour
- 3/4 cup buttermilk
- 2 eggs
- 2 tablespoons Vegetable oil

Dressing
- 8 tablespoons butter (1 stick)
- 3 medium onion, chopped
- 4 stalks celery, chopped
- 1 1/2 teaspoons dried sage
- 1 teaspoon poultry seasoning
- 3/4 teaspoon salt
- 1/2 teaspoon pepper
- 3 pieces toast, crumbled
- 1/2 cup milk
- 3 eggs, lightly beaten
- 2 to 2 1/2 cups chicken stock or broth
- 2 tablespoons butter

SOUTHERN CORNBREAD DRESSING!

Directions:

·Preheat oven to 400 degrees.

·In a medium bowl, stir together all ingredients for cornbread. Pour into a lightly greased 9-inch cast iron pan or a 9-inch baking pan. Bake for 20 to 25 minutes. Before using, crumble into small pieces.

·Heat butter over medium heat in a large pan. Add celery and onion and cook until soft. Add sage, poultry seasoning, salt, and pepper to onion mixture.

·In a large bowl combine crumbled cornbread and toast.

·Whisk together milk and eggs and add to bowl. Stir in 2 cups of chicken broth.

·Stir in onion mixture. Mixture should be very moist. Add more broth if necessary.

·Transfer to a greased baking dish. Cut butter into small slivers and scatter on top of dressing.

Bake at 350 degrees for 30 minutes, or until it turns light brown on top.

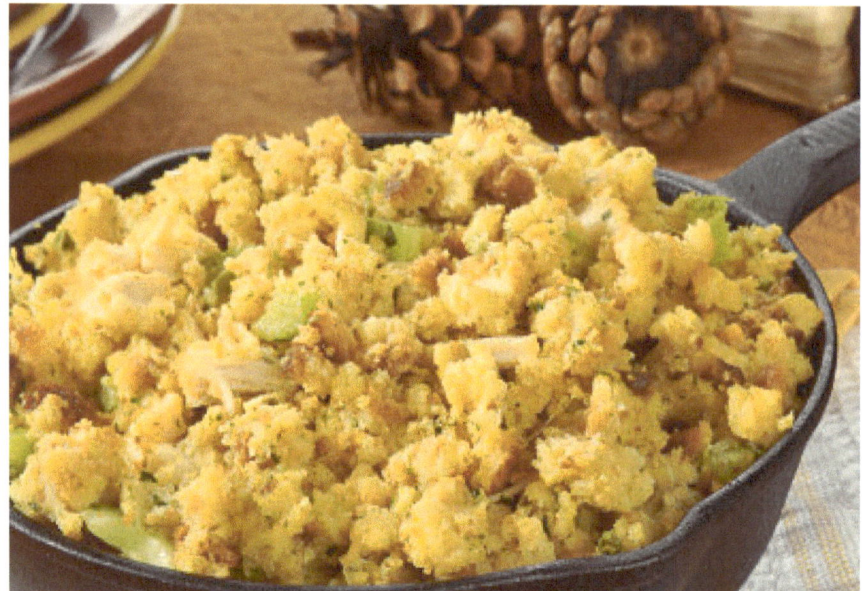

Best keep secret for Soulful Cornbread dressing use extra pinch of black pepper to get a spicy taste and add a pinch of Slap Yo Mamma Cajun Seasoning to taste. To make it creamy use a can of Campbell's Celery Soup along with chicken broth!

Sweet Candied Potatoes!

Ingredients:

- 1 1/2 pounds sweet potatoes
- 4 tablespoons butter
- 1 cup brown sugar, packed, light or dark
- 2 small cinnamon sticks, about 2 1/2 inches in length
- Pinch of ground cinnamon
- 1/2 cup orange juice or pineapple juice (or some people like to use apple juice)

Directions:

1. Peel the sweet potatoes and slice into rounds about 1/4-inch thick. If one or both of the potatoes are very wide, cut in half lengthwise before slicing.
2. In a large heavy skillet (preferably a seasoned iron skillet) or Dutch oven over medium-low heat, melt the butter.
3. Add the brown sugar, cinnamon sticks, pinch of cinnamon and orange juice to the melted butter and bring to a simmer.
4. Add the sweet potato slices to the juice mixture. Cover and simmer, stirring and turning frequently, for about 25 to 30 minutes.
5. Remove the cover and let the syrup cook down, taking care not to let it burn. Gently turn the potatoes from time to time to keep them coated.
6. Transfer to a serving dish. As a variation, toast a handful of pecan halves

in a dry skillet over medium heat until lightly browned and aromatic. Add them to the glazed sweet potatoes and toss to coat.

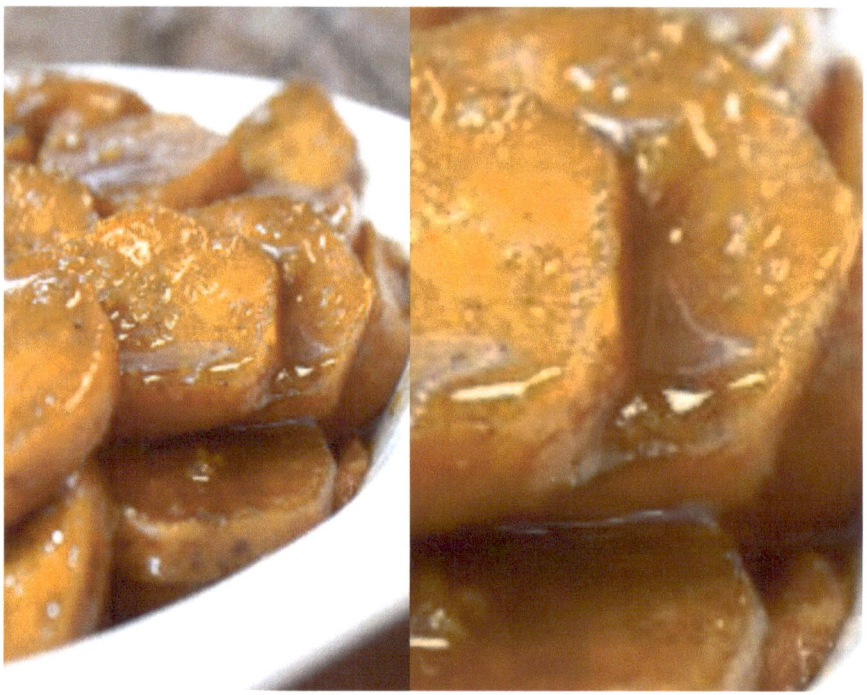

Creole Roast Turkey!

Ingredients:

- 1 turkey (14 to 16 pounds)
- 1 cup butter, softened
- 3 tablespoons Creole seasoning -Like Slap Ya Mamma Cajun Seasoning
- 2 table spoon Black Pepper
- 1 tablespoon sage
- Whole cloves of garlic and
- 1 quartered onion
- ½ cup chopped celery
- 1 apple quartered

Directions:

- Preheat oven to 400°. Season turkey cavity with 1 tbsp. of the sage and 1 tablespoon of creole seasoning/Slap Ya Mamma seasoning and 1 tablespoon of black pepper to taste. Next sprinkle whole body of turkey with the rest of the creole seasoning and black pepper. Next placed quartered onion, apple and celery along with garlic cloves into turkey cavity. Tuck wings under turkey; (or place aluminum foil over each turkey wing tip. Next, tie drumsticks together. Place on a rack in a shallow roasting pan, breast side up. In a small bowl, beat butter and Creole seasoning (or Slap Ya Mamma Cajun Seasoning); rub over turkey. Roast, uncovered, 20 minutes.

·Reduce oven setting to 325°. Roast 3-1/4 to 3-3/4 hours longer or until a thermometer inserted in thickest part of thigh reads 170°-175°. (Cover loosely with foil if turkey browns too quickly.)

Remove turkey from oven; tent with foil. Let stand 20 minutes before carving. Skim fat from pan drippings; serve drippings with turkey and vegetable mixture.

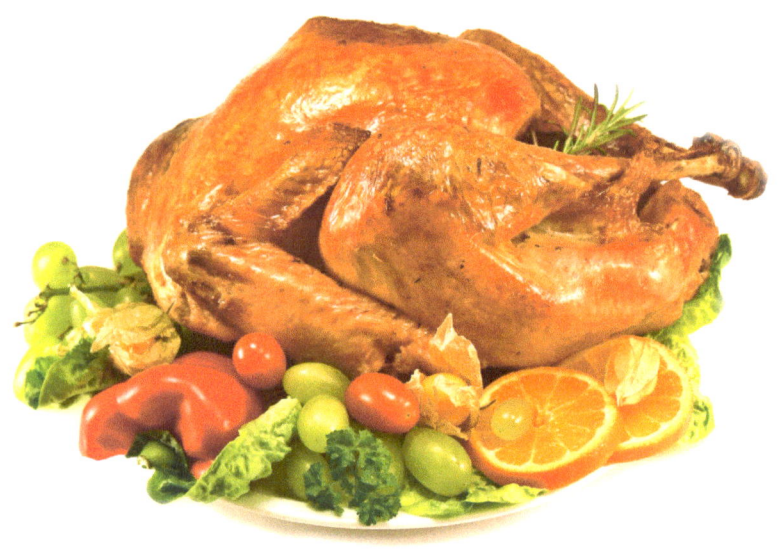

Hickory Smoked Bacon Collard Greens!

Ingredients:

- 2 pounds collard greens
  - 4 thick-sliced bacon strips, chopped
  - 1 cup chopped sweet onion
  - 5 cups reduced-sodium chicken broth
  - 1 teaspoon Slap Ya Mamma Cajun Seasoning
  - 1/2 teaspoon garlic powder or 2 cloves garlic, chopped
  - 1/4 teaspoon hickory flavored liquid smoke or just plain liquid smoke
  - 1/4 teaspoon of brown sugar
  - 1/4 teaspoon crushed red pepper flakes

Directions:

- Trim thick stems from collard greens; coarsely chop leaves. In a Dutch oven, sauté bacon for 3 minutes. Add onion; cook 8-9 minutes longer or until onion is tender and bacon is crisp. Add greens; cook just until wilted.
  - Stir in remaining ingredients. Bring to a boil. Reduce heat; cover and simmer for 45-50 minutes or until greens are tender.

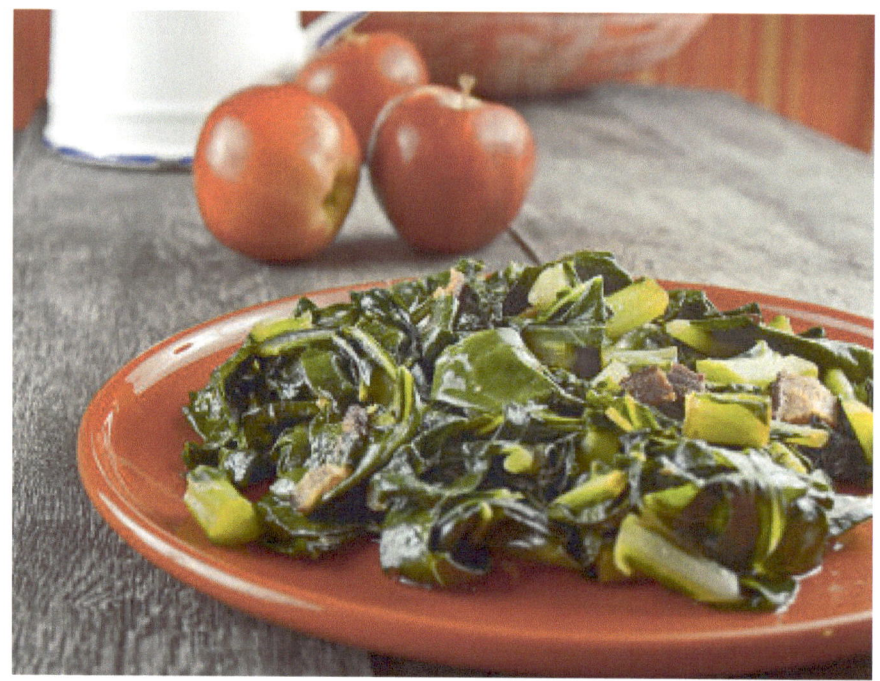

Collard greens and bacon!

Angel Biscuits!

Ingredients:

- 1/2 cup warm water (100°F to 110°F)
- 1 (1/4-oz.) pkg. active dry yeast (2 1/4 tsp.)
- 1 teaspoon plus 3 Tbsp. granulated sugar, divided
- 5 cups all-purpose flour
- 1 tablespoon baking powder
- 1 1/2 teaspoons salt
- 1 teaspoon baking soda
- 1/2 cup cold salted butter, cubed
- 1/2 cup cold shortening, cubed
- 2 cups whole buttermilk
- 6 tablespoons salted butter, melted and divided

Directions:

- Stir together warm water, yeast, and 1 teaspoon of the sugar in a small bowl. Let stand 5 minutes.

  - Stir together flour, baking powder, salt, baking soda, and remaining 3 tablespoons sugar in a large bowl; cut cold butter and cold shortening into flour mixture with a pastry blender or 2 forks until crumbly. Add yeast mixture and buttermilk to flour mixture, stirring just until dry ingredients are moistened. Cover bowl with plastic wrap; chill at least 2 hours or up to 5 days.

·Preheat oven to 400°F. Turn dough out onto a lightly floured surface and knead 3 or 4 times. Gently roll into a 1/2-inch-thick circle, and fold in half; repeat. Gently roll to 1/2-inch thickness; cut with a 2-inch round cutter. Re-roll remaining scraps and cut with cutter. Place rounds with sides touching in a 12-inch cast-iron skillet or on a parchment paper-lined baking sheet. (If using a 12-inch skillet, place remaining biscuits in a 10-inch skillet or on a baking sheet.) Brush biscuits with 3 tablespoons of the melted butter.

·Bake in preheated oven until golden, 15 to 20 minutes. Brush with remaining 3 tablespoons melted butter and serve hot out the oven.

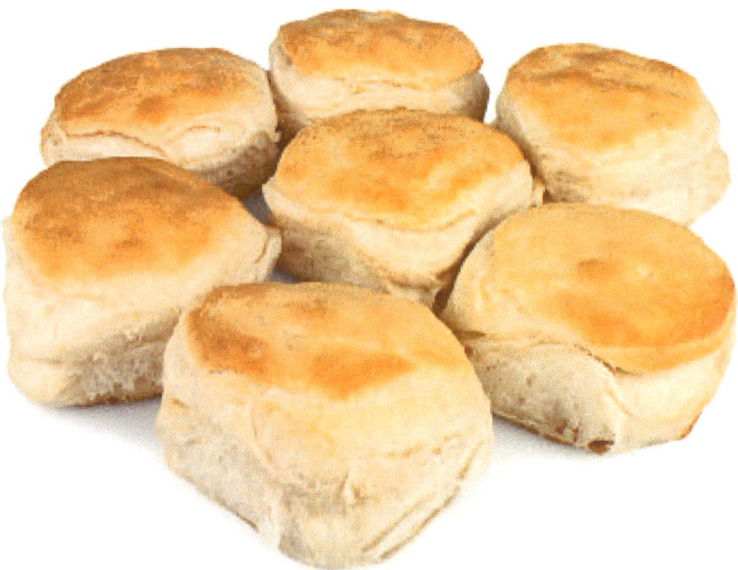

Angel Biscuits!

Pineapple Brown Sugar Glazed Ham!

Ingredients:

- 1 fully cooked bone-in ham (7 to 9 pounds)
- 1 can (20 ounces) crushed pineapple, undrained
- 1 cup packed brown sugar
- 1 tablespoon Dijon mustard
- 1/4 teaspoon ground cloves
- 1 can whole pineapple slices for garnish *optional*

Directions:

- Preheat oven to 325°. Place ham on a rack in a shallow roasting pan. Using a sharp knife, score surface of ham with 1/2-in.-deep cuts in a diamond pattern. Cover and bake 1-1/2 hours.
- In a small bowl, mix remaining ingredients. Spread over ham, pressing mixture into cuts. Bake ham, uncovered, 30-60 minutes longer.

THE SWEET PEPPER CAJUN! TASTY SOULFUL FOOD COOKBOOK!

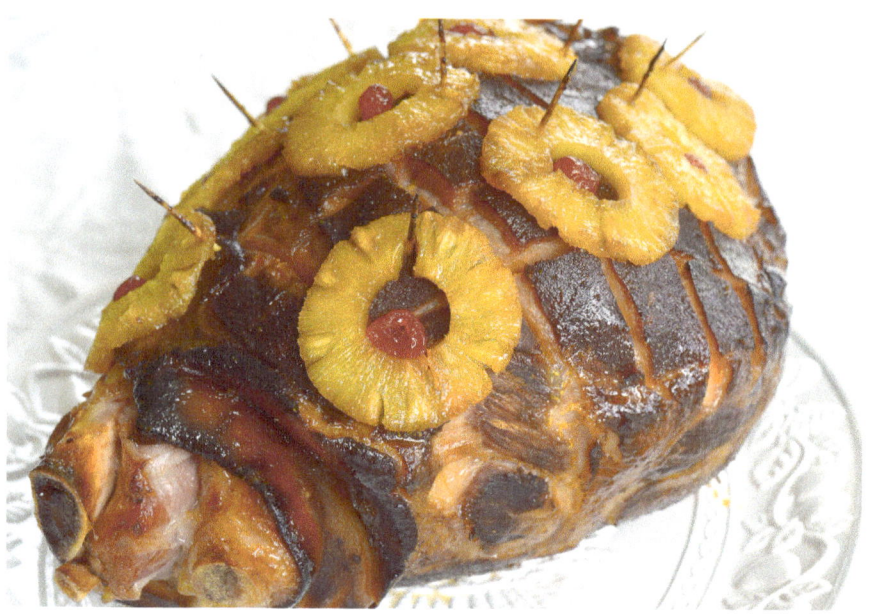

PINEAPPLE BROWN SUGAR GLAZED HAM!

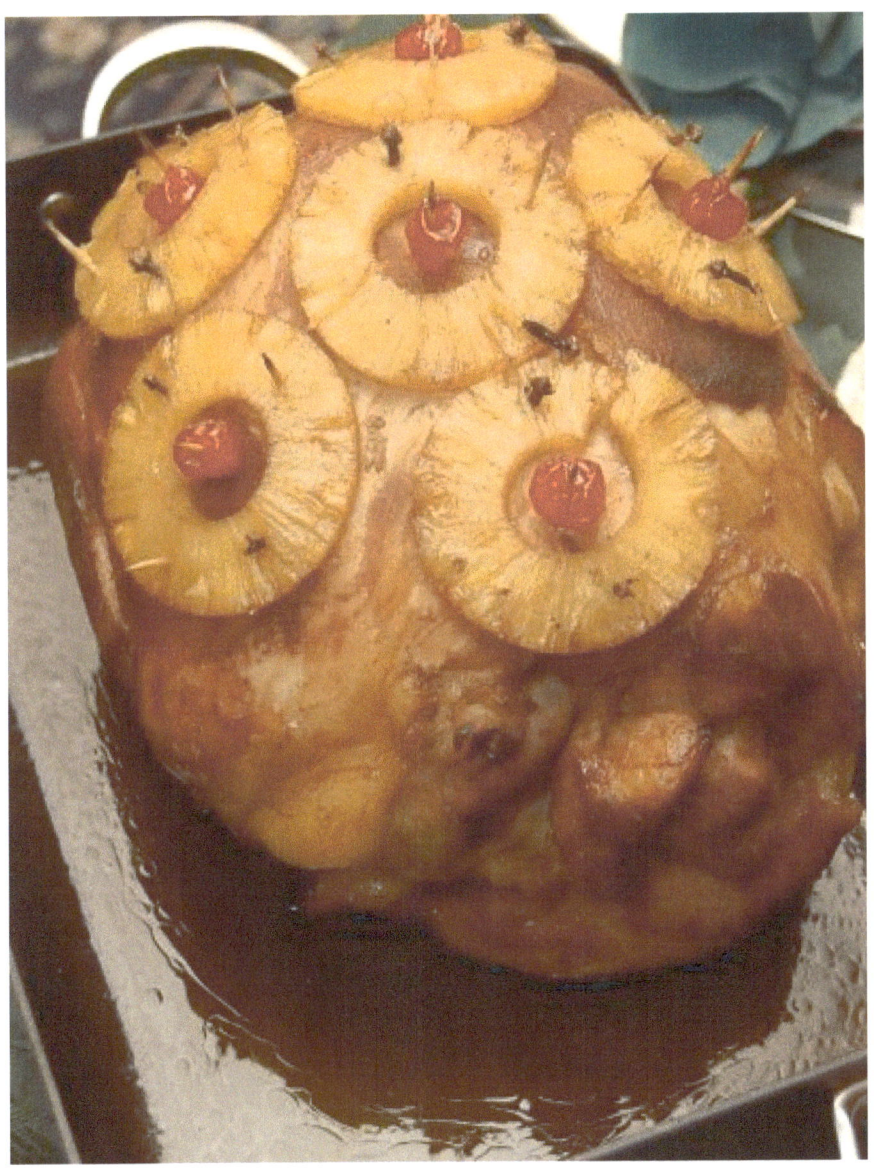

Creamy Cheesy Scalloped Potatoes!

Ingredients;
- 2 tablespoons butter
- 5 lbs. Yukon Gold Potatoes scrubbed and partially cooked in the microwave 4-6 minutes (this will shorten the cooking time in the oven.
- 2 cups heavy cream
- 2 5.6 oz. ea. packages Boursin Cheese, garlic & herb (can find this cheese at Wal-Mart & Target)
- ¾ teaspoon kosher salt
- ½ teaspoon ground black pepper
- Grated Parmesan for garnish

Directions:

1. Preheat oven to 400-degree F.
2. Spray any 8 x 11-inch casserole dish with non-stick spray and dot the bottom with butter. Place it in the oven until butter melts then remove the pan from the oven.
3. In a medium saucepan, heat heavy cream, (make sure milk does scorch) add the Boursin cheese, salt and pepper over medium-low heat just until the cheese melts and stir until mixture is smooth. Set mixture aside until ready to use.
4. Slice the partially cooked potatoes with a mandolin (if available) into 3/16" slices (a food process works fine also with their chopping thin slice blade). Place the sliced potatoes in a large bowl and pour the cheese/cream

CREAMY CHEESY SCALLOPED POTATOES!

mixture over all them.

(*Next use a tong to pick up potato slices to layer in their casserole dish.)

5. Pick up several potato slices and place them in the casserole dish. Organize the slices into a small stack then place them vertically along the side of the dish or in a circular shape, you decide. Repeat with all the potato slices, placing them where needed. The potatoes should be tightly packed.

6. Pour the excess cheese/cream mixture over the potatoes until the mixture comes up almost to the top.

7. Cover the dish with foil and place it on a foil-lined baking sheet pan. Place the dish in the preheated oven and bake 30 minutes. Remove the foil covering from the dish and bake another 30 minutes then sprinkle grated Parmesan over the potatoes. Bake 15-30 more minutes until the top is golden brown, the middle is bubbly, and potatoes are cooked through. Total cook time is 75-90 minutes.

8. Remove potatoes from the oven, all to rest 5-10 minutes before serving.

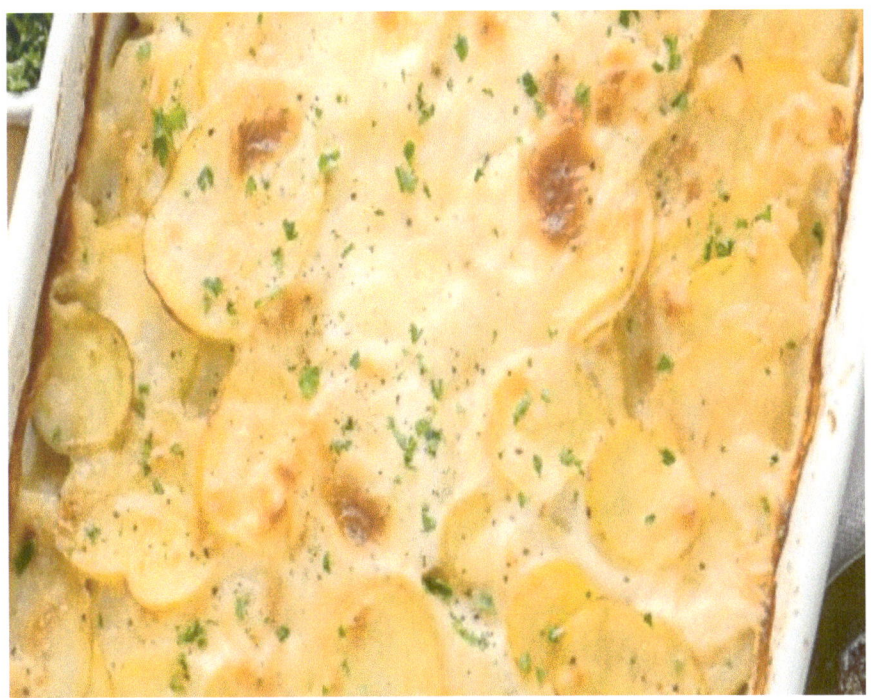

Roasted Holiday Veggies!

Ingredients:

1 pound of Brussels sprouts, trimmed and halved
2 large carrots, peeled and sliced into 1/2" pieces
2 tbsp. extra-virgin olive oil
1 tbsp. balsamic vinegar
1 tsp. chopped rosemary leaves
1 tsp. chopped thyme leaves
½ teaspoon Kosher salt
½ tablespoon Slap Ya Mamma Cajun seasoning
½ tablespoon Freshly ground black pepper
1/2 cup toasted pecans
1/2 cup dried cranberries

Directions:

1. Preheat oven to 400°. Scatter vegetables on a large baking sheet. Toss with oil, balsamic vinegar, rosemary, and thyme. Season with salt and pepper.
2. Bake for 20 to 25 minutes, until the vegetable are tender, shaking the pan halfway through.

Before serving, toss roasted vegetables with pecans and cranberries.

Butternut Squash & Andouille Dressing!

Ingredients:

1 small butternut squash (about 1 1/2 pounds, diced
   3 tbsp. extra-virgin olive oil, divided
   kosher salt
   Freshly ground black pepper
   8 oz. andouille, sliced 1/4"-thick
   1 large yellow onion, chopped
   3 celery stalks, chopped
   10 c. torn baguette or other crusty bread, dried overnight
   1/4 c. freshly chopped sage
   2 tbsp. freshly chopped parsley, plus more for serving
   2 large eggs
   3 c. low-sodium vegetable or chicken broth, divided
   4 tbsp. butter, cut into 1/2" pieces

Directions:

1. Preheat oven to 425°. Toss squash with 2 tablespoons olive oil and season with salt and pepper on a rimmed baking sheet. Roast until golden and tender, 20 to 25 minutes, then reduce heat to 350°.

2. Heat remaining tablespoon olive oil in a large skillet over medium heat. Add andouille and cook, stirring often, until golden and crisp, about 4

minutes, then transfer to a plate using a slotted spoon. Add onion and celery to skillet and season with salt and pepper. Cook, stirring often, until vegetables are tender, 6 to 8 minutes. Transfer vegetables to a large bowl and add baguette pieces, sage, parsley, roasted squash, and andouille and toss to combine.

3.In a separate medium bowl, whisk together eggs and 2 cups broth. Pour over bread mixture and toss until evenly moistened, adding more broth ¼ cup at a time until baguette pieces seem hydrated (you might not use it all).

4.Transfer mixture to prepared baking dish and dot with butter. Cover dish with foil and bake until a knife inserted in the center of the stuffing comes out warm, 30 to 35 minutes. Increase oven to 450° and continue baking until top is deeply golden, 15 to 20 minutes more.

5.Let rest for 10 minutes, garnish with parsley and serve.

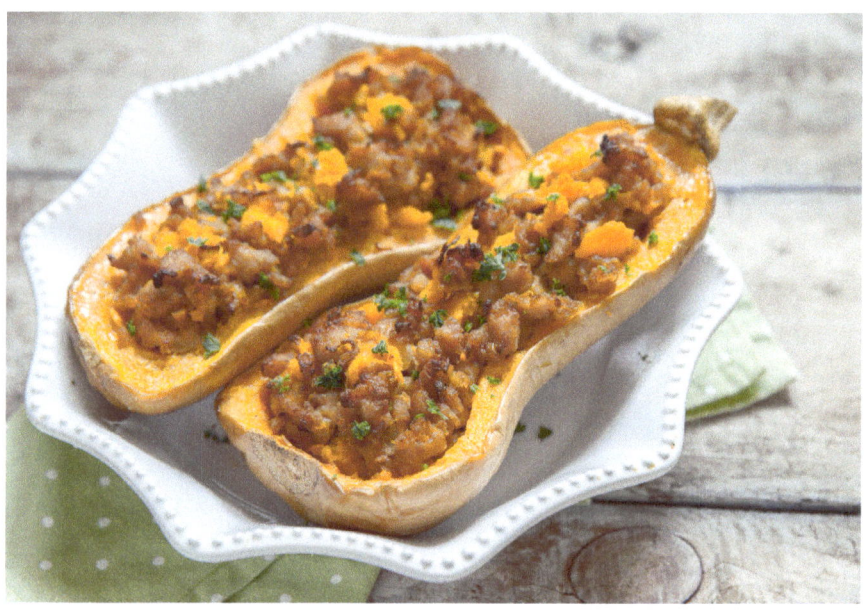

Your presentation will be unique when you serve your Butternut Squash & Andouille Dressing in the shell!

Cranberry Salad Mold!

Ingredients:

- 1 (8-oz.) can crushed pineapple in syrup
  - Boiling water
  - 1 (3-oz.) package raspberry-flavored gelatin
  - 1 (14-oz.) can whole-berry cranberry sauce
  - 1 cup* drained mandarin oranges* optional blueberries garnish optional
  - 1 teaspoon orange zest

Directions:

Drain syrup from pineapple into a 2-cup measuring cup. Add boiling water to equal 1 1/4 cups. Transfer to a large bowl. Dissolve gelatin in hot syrup mixture; chill 1 hour and 30 minutes or until partially set. Fold in cranberry sauce, oranges, zest, and crushed pineapple. Pour into 1 (4-cup) mold, and chill 2 hours or until set.

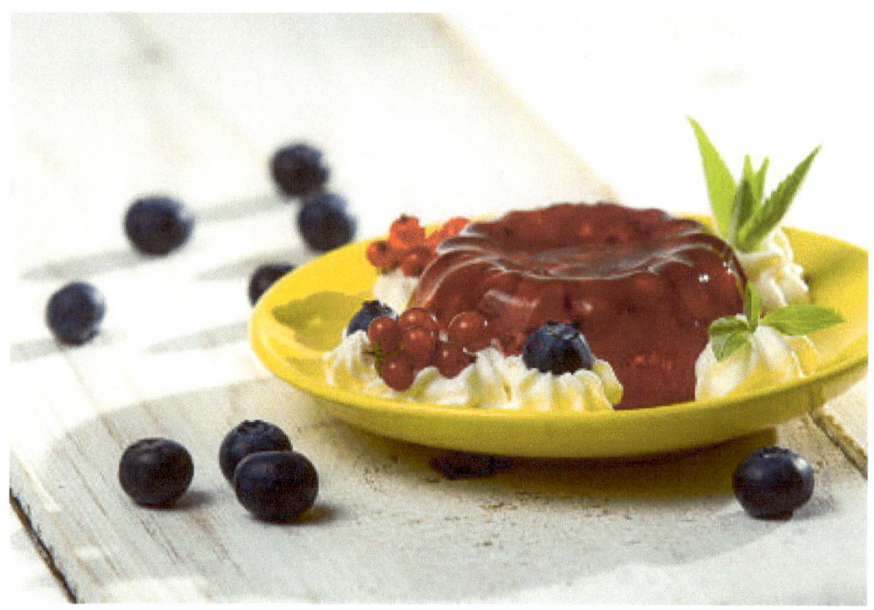

Cranberry Pineapple Melody!

Ingredients:

- 4 cups fresh or frozen cranberries (14 oz.)
  - 3/4 cup packed light brown sugar
  - 1/2 cup fresh orange juice (from 2 oranges)
  - 1 cup peeled and chopped Bartlett pears (about 2 small pears)
  - 1 cup chopped fresh pineapple (from 1 pineapple)
  - 1/2 cup thinly sliced celery (from 2 stalks)
  - 1/2 cup chopped toasted pecans

Directions:

1. Bring the cranberries, brown sugar, and orange juice to a boil in a large saucepan over medium-high, stirring often. Reduce heat to medium-low, and simmer, stirring occasionally, until cranberries pop and mixture thickens, 12 to 15 minutes. Remove from heat, and cool to room temperature, about 30 minutes.

2. Stir in the Bartlett pears, pineapple, celery, and pecans. Transfer to a serving bowl; cover and chill salad. Serves 4 to 24.

Mamma's Million Dollar Pound Cake!

For Best Results preheat oven to 300 degrees before you begin and soften butter to room temperature for at least 30 minutes. Also use all purpose flour and shift the dry ingredients together prior to mixing, shifting together twice makes for a smooth cake.*

Ingredients:

- 1 pound butter, softened
  - 3 cups sugar
  - 6 large eggs
  - 4 cups all-purpose flour
  - ½ teaspoon baking powder
  - 1.4 teaspoon of salt
  - 3/4 cup milk
  - 1 teaspoon lemon extract
  - 1 teaspoon vanilla extract

Directions:

Step 1

Beat butter at medium speed with an electric mixer until creamy. (The butter will become a lighter yellow color; this is an important step, as the job of the mixer is to incorporate air into the butter so the cake will rise. It will take 1 to 7 minutes, depending on the power of your mixer.) Gradually add sugar, beating at medium speed until light and fluffy. (Again, the times will vary, and butter will turn to a fluffy white.) Add eggs, 1 at a time, beating just until yellow yolk disappears.

Step 2

Add flour mixture (*all mixed dry ingredients) to creamed mixture alternately with milk, beginning and ending with flour. Beat at low speed just until blended after each addition. (The batter should be smooth, and bits of flour should be well incorporated; to rid batter of lumps, stir gently with a rubber spatula.) Stir in extracts.

Step 3

Pour into a greased and floured 10-inch tube pan. (Use vegetable shortening or butter to grease the pan, getting every nook and cranny covered. Sprinkle a light coating of flour over the greased surface.)

Step 4

Bake at 300° for 1 hour and 40 minutes or until a long wooden pick inserted in center comes out clean. Cool in pan on a wire rack 10 to 15 minutes. Remove from pan, and cool completely on a wire rack.

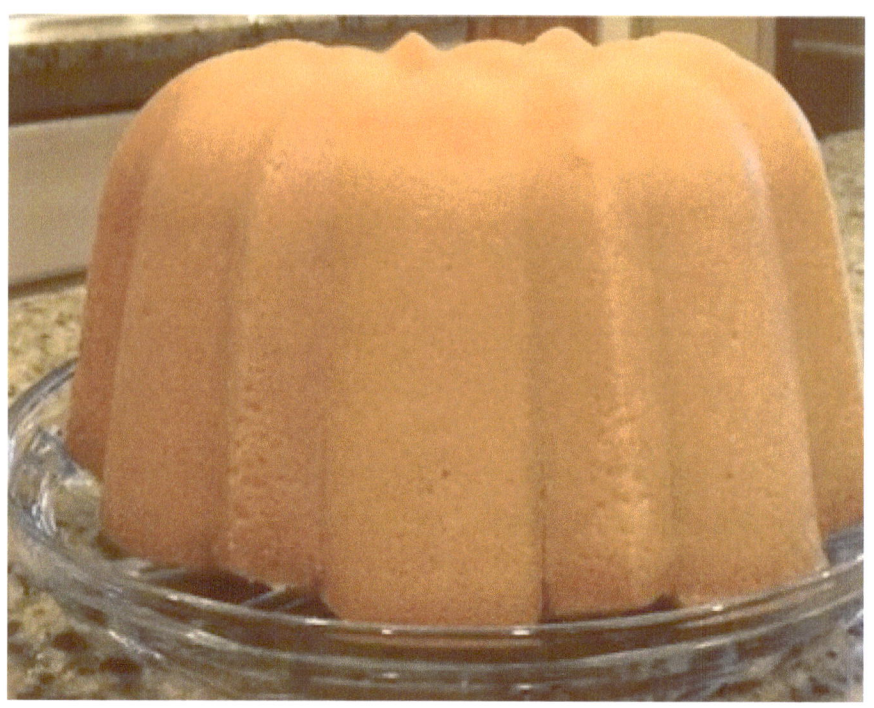

Mamma's Million Dollar Pound Cake!

MAMMA'S MILLION DOLLAR POUND CAKE!

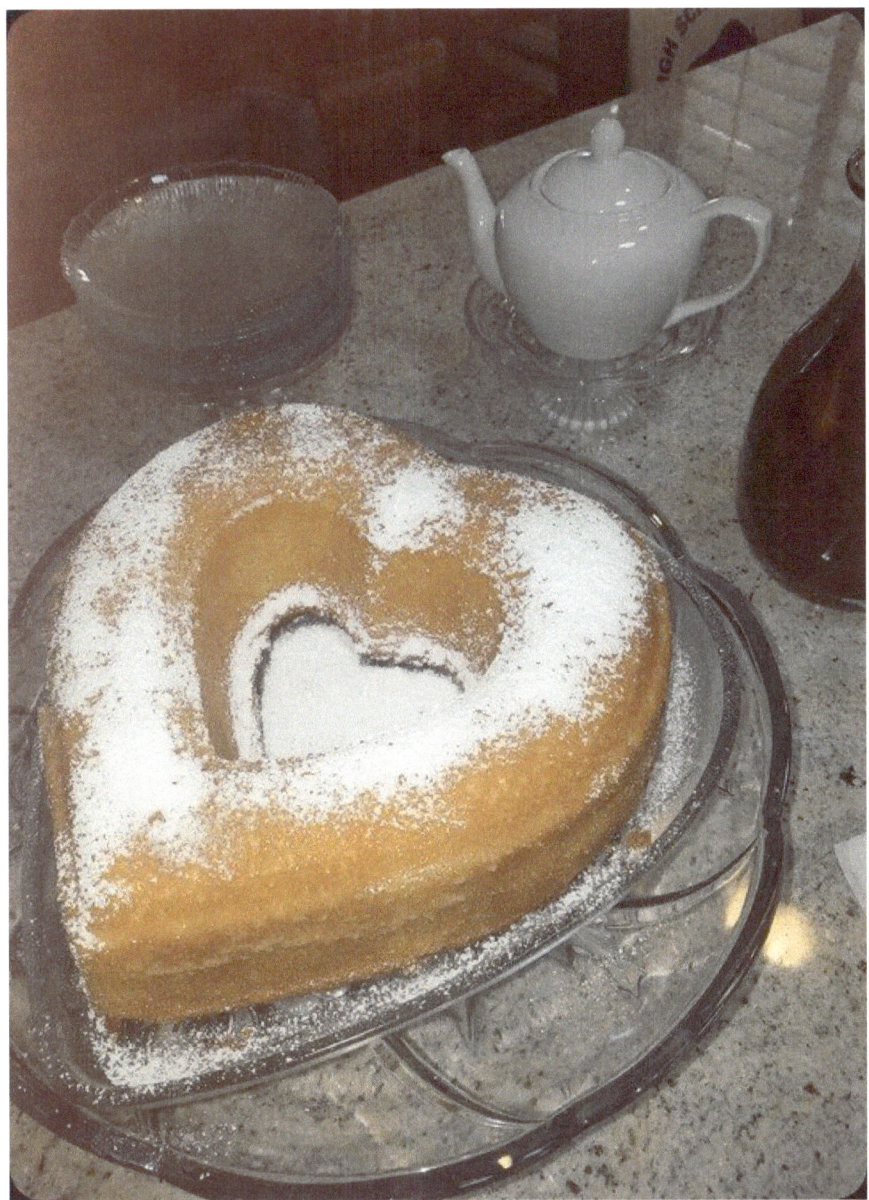

This my favorite pan to make this Pound Cake in, I also have a beautiful heart-shaped cake plate to place it on. I love this effect and hope you do too.

30 Minutes Dinner Rolls!

Ingredients:

- 1 cup warm tap water
- 1/3 cup oil
- 1/4 cup sugar
- 2 tablespoons yeast
- 1/2 teaspoon salt
- 1 egg *beaten*
- 1 tablespoon softened butter
- 3 to 4 cups all-purpose flour *I used closer to 3*
- 1/8 cup milk *room temperature*

Directions:

1. Preheat oven to 400 degrees.
2. In a large bowl, combine 1 cup water, oil, sugar, and yeast. Let sit until yeast is bubbly (about 8 minutes). Stir in beaten egg softened butter and salt.
3. With a stand mixer or by hand, add flour, one cup at a time until you have a soft dough that isn't sticky. Knead by hand 10 minutes or 5 minutes with a stand mixer.
4. Divide dough into 18 even pieces, and form into balls. Place in a greased pan and cover with parchment paper. Let dough rest at least ten minutes

before baking in the oven. *Smear tops of finished hot rolls with melted and garlic for an added flavor.

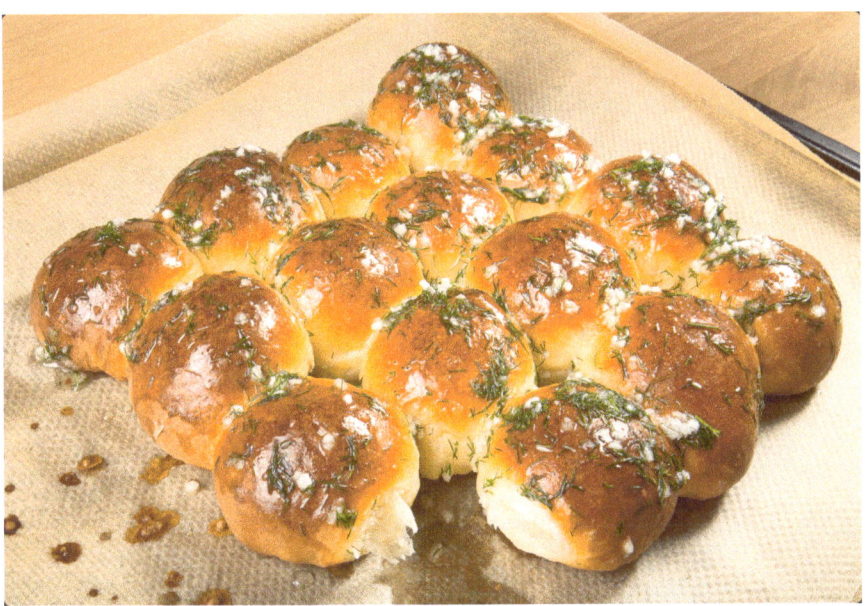

Holidays Time For Family & Friends!

Come join us, grab a seat, fill a bowl, and take a taste of our scrumptious food. We believe food is our common ground and in flavor do we trust! Any Season!

There's an old saying... "Good friends are so very hard to find, and I'm am so grateful that you are mine." This is for you... All of my friends. Thank you.

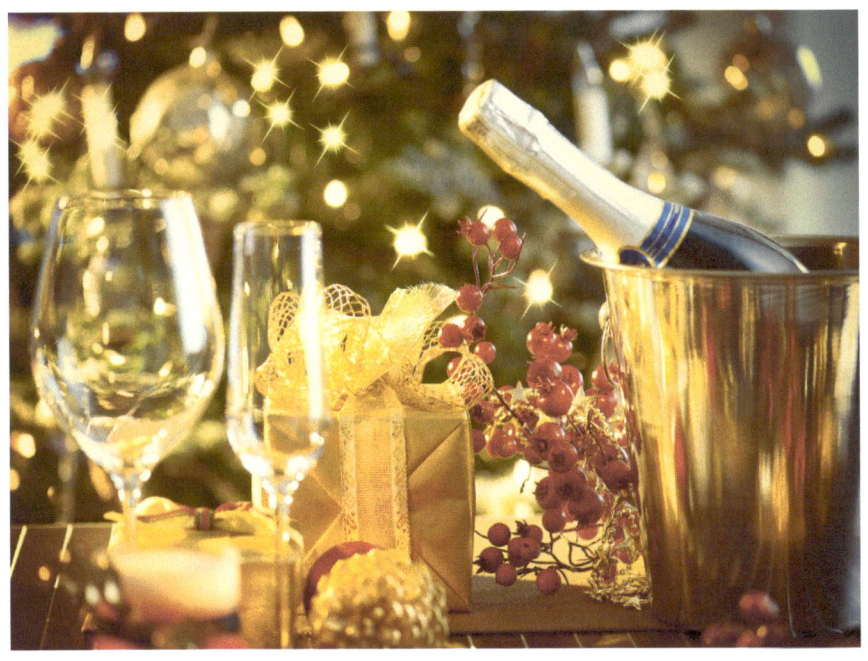

Traditional Southern New Year's New Dinner!

**Traditional Southern
New Year's New Dinner!**

**Beyond Black-Eyed Peas!
Good Luck Is Your Destiny!**

~Menu~

**Black-Eyed Peas
Rice
Collard Greens or Mixed Greens
Silver Scaled Fish
Golden Brown Cornbread
Good Luck Long Noodle Creamy Cajun Pasta
Traditional New Year's Roasted Pork
New Year's Good Luck Pound Cake**

* * *

Meanings of each food Dish.

Black-Eyed Peas ~ Prosperity and Abundance is their meaning, along with Good Luck. That's why you must serve Black-Eyed Peas, for your New Year's Dinner so that you can have good luck throughout the year.

Rice is always served along with Black-Eyed Peas. **Rice represents abundance**.

Greens ~ **Money**! The color of money is represented in the **Collard Greens, Turnip Greens, Mustard Greens, Chard, Spinach, and Kale**, as well as in the green color of Green Cabbage.

Pork or Pig is of course the Main Course of any Traditional Southern New Year's Dinner, because the **Pig symbolizes progress or moving forward**.

Round cakes or pies served at New Year's Dinner also **symbolizes mone**y, their round shape symbolizes **coin money**.

Silver Fish - Serving Silver-scaled fish at Southern New Year's Dinner is done because it too represents abundance and wealth. Its silver color represents the **wealth of Silver** and the fact that Fish swim, **symbolizes money swimmin**g through your household abundantly during the coming New Year.

Golden Brown Cornbread, as the name implies it represent the **wealth of Gold**. Gold's value never needs to be explain.

This New Year I added something New to New Years' Dinner – **Long uncut Noodles**. I'm serving them Cream Cajun Noodle Style. Why the long noodle? In many cultures, eating uncut noodles without breaking them **ensures good health** throughout the coming year. Therefore add some good health to your New Year's Good Luck Dinner!

Here's Wishing Everyone A Very Happy New Year's Dinner!

Traditional New Year's Pork Roast!

Ingredients:

- 1 (5-6 pound) pork butt
  - 6 cloves garlic, chopped
  - 1/2 cup green onions, sliced
  - 1/4 tsp cayenne pepper
  - 1/4 teaspoon onion powder
  - 1/4 teaspoon garlic powder
  - 1/8 teaspoon black pepper
  - 1/4 teaspoon rubbed sage
  - 1/8 tsp dried basil
  - 2 tsp Slap Ya Mamma Cajun Seasoning
  - 1 tsp red pepper flakes
  - 1/4 cup vegetable oil
  - 1 onion, quartered
  - 2 ribs celery, chopped
  - 1 carrot, chopped

Directions:

Preheat oven to 375 degrees F. In a small mixing bowl combine garlic, green onions, cayenne pepper, rubbed sage, basil, garlic powder onion powder, Slap Ya Mamma Cajun seasoning, and peppers. Using a paring knife, pierce 1-inch holes evenly across the roast (approximately 8) and fill each cavity with an equal amount of the mixture. Season the roast completely on the outside. In a 12-quart Dutch oven, heat oil over medium-high heat. Brown roast on all sides. Add quartered onions, celery and carrot. Cover the pot, place in oven and bake until fork tender, approximately 2½ - 3 hours. When the roast is tender, remove the cover and brown 15-20 minutes. Leftovers of this meat makes great sandwiches.

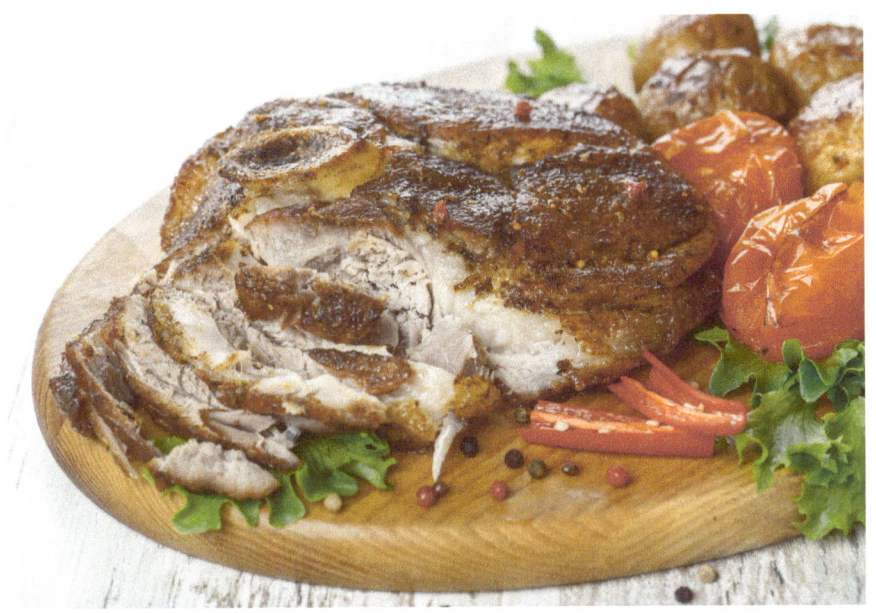

Bone in Pork Shoulder!

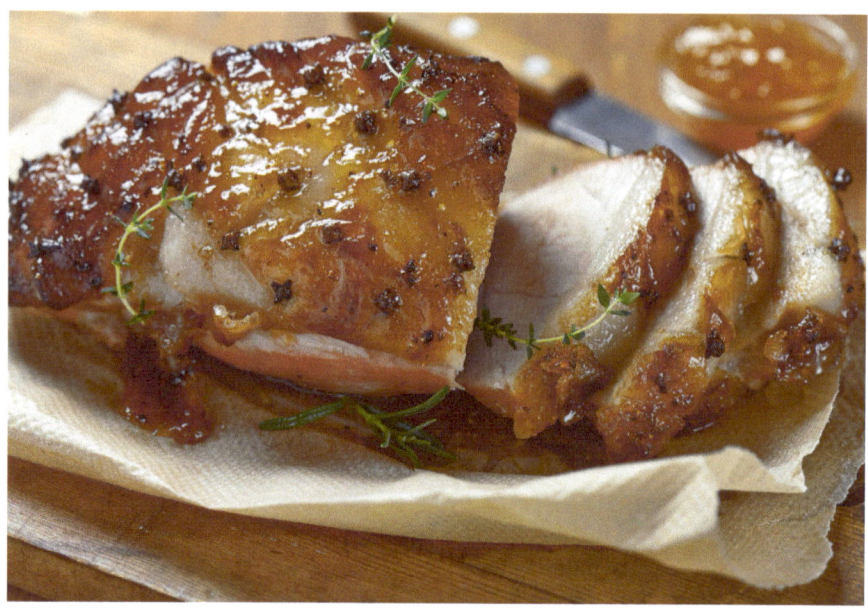

Pork Loin Roast!

If you love Pork Loin Roast instead of a Pork Shoulder Roast your cooking time for the Pork Loin Roast is 25 minutes per pound or until the internal temperature reaches 145 degrees. Be sure to baste the Pork Loin Roast while cooking.

New Year's Good Luck Long Noodle Creamy Cajun Pasta!

New Year's Good Luck Long Noodle Creamy Cajun Pasta

Ingredients:
- 8 ounces linguine or thick spaghetti cooked al dente
- 2 teaspoons Slap Ya Mamma Cajun seasoning
- 2 tablespoons butter
- 1 tablespoon flour
- 2 tablespoon olive oil
- ½ cup diced onion
- ½ cup diced bell pepper
- 1 thinly sliced green onion
- 1/2 cup heavy whipping cream
- 1/2 cup chicken broth
- ½ cup mozzarella cheese
- ¼ cup Parmesan
- ½ cup cream cheese (4 oz of Philadelphia Cheese)
- 2 tablespoons chopped sun-dried tomatoes
- ¼ teaspoon salt
- ¼ teaspoon dried basil
- 1/8 teaspoon ground black pepper

- 1/8 teaspoon garlic powder
- 1/8 onion powder

Directions:

- In a large skillet add olive oil and onions and bell pepper cook until tender
- In a separate skillet (or the same skillet as onions and bell pepper if you are comfortable using one skillet — *If using one skillet move the sauté onions and bell pepper to one side of the skillet, on the other side and on lower heat to medium), stir in butter or margarine until melted and add the flour until it dissolves. Do not scorch flour.
- Reduce heat, add heavy cream,
- Slowly add Cream Cheese, mozzarella cheese, Parmesan cheese slow add chicken broth as sauce thickens
- Add tomatoes, basil, Slap Ya Mamma seasoning salt, garlic powder, onion powder black pepper and heat through.
- Pour over hot linguine or thick spaghetti Noodles and toss with Parmesan cheese.

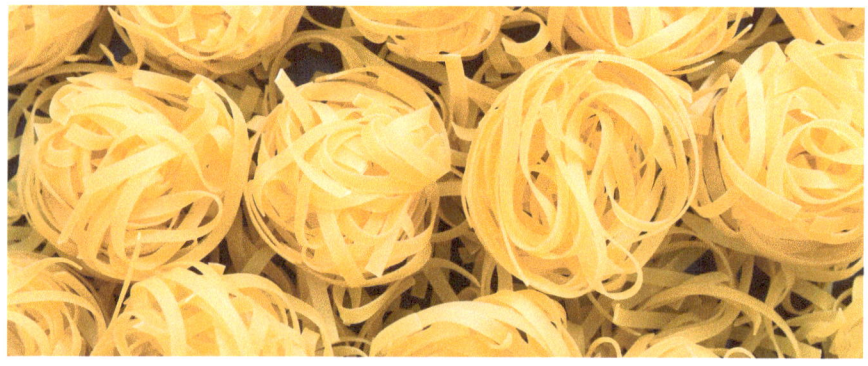

Long linguine or thick spaghetti are excellent for this dish!

Smoky Black-Eyed Peas!

Ingredients:

- 1-pound dried black-eyed peas
- 4 ounces smoked turkey (smoked turkey wings, turkey are excellent to use)
- 1 large whole onion
- 1 small diced onion
- 3 to 4 cloves garlic
- ½ teaspoon liquid smoke
- 2 ribs celery (diced)
- 1/2 red bell pepper (diced)
- 1/2 green bell pepper (diced)
- 2 teaspoons Cajun seasoning mixture (or a seasoning salt blend)
- 1/2 teaspoon kosher salt (or to taste)
- ¼ teaspoon Slap Ya Mamma Cajun seasoning.
- 1/4 teaspoon pepper
- Optional: cayenne pepper (to taste

Directions:

1. Gather the ingredients.
2. Rinse the black-eyed peas and pick them over, removing any damaged peas or small stones. Put them in a large Dutch oven and cover with water to

a depth of about 3 inches above the peas. Cover the pan.

3. Following package directions, soak the black-eyed peas overnight or boil for 2 minutes and then let them stand for 1 hour. Drain the peas.

4. Using Large Stock Pot add the smoke turkey and cover with water and bring to a slow boil.

5. Peel the onion and cut it in half. If you are using whole cloves press them into the onion skin as it makes for easy find when you get ready to serve.

6. Peel and mince the garlic.

7. Place a heavy skillet over medium heat and sauté the diced onion until lightly browned. Add the garlic and continue to cook for 1 minute longer.

8. Meanwhile, dice celery, and the red and green bell peppers, if using. Peel and cut onion in half.

9. Transfer drained peas to pot with slowing boiling turkey. Add the celery, the red and green bell pepper (if using), add the halved onion, and cooked onions, and the Cajun seasoning blend. Make sure water in pot covers peas. Add the liquid smoke.

10. Simmer the peas for about 1 1/2 to 2 1/2 hours, or until the peas and vegetables are tender. Check the peas occasionally to make sure it has water and add a little more water if necessary. Taste and season with more Slap Ya Mamma Cajun seasoning, black pepper, and hot pepper, as desired.

11. About 20 minutes before the peas are ready, cook the rice following the package directions. Keep the rice warm until serving time.

SMOKY BLACK-EYED PEAS!

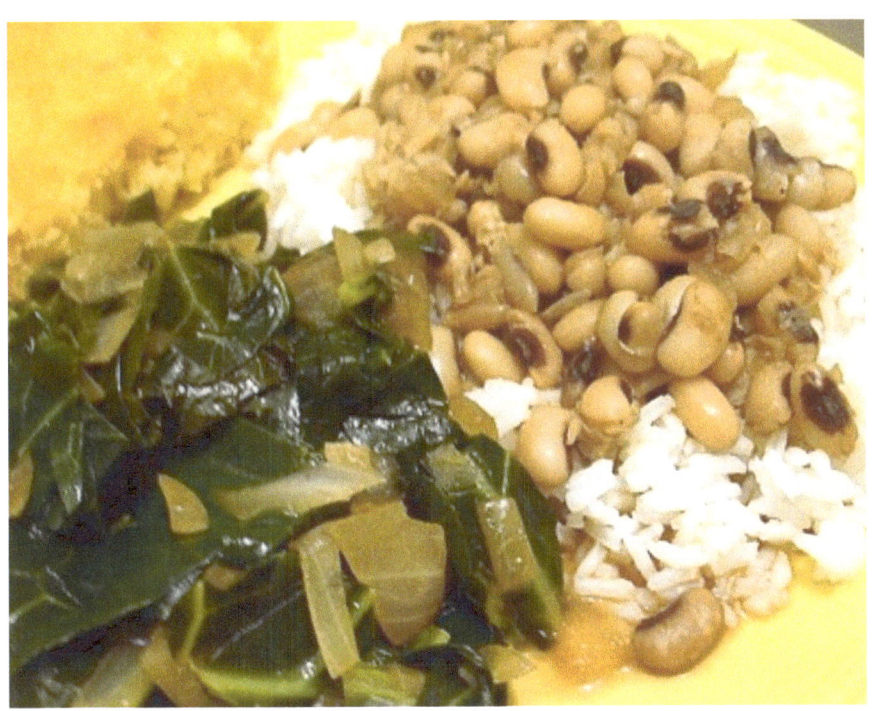

Baked Silver Fish!

Ingredients:

Serves 4
- 3 Silver Fish (scaled, & gutted) or filet
- 4 sprig Italian Flat-Leaf Parsley
- 1/4 teaspoon of Marjoram
- 1/4 teaspoon Sage
- 4 sprig Fresh Basil
- 6 clove peeled Garlic
- 3 Large Lemon
- 2 tablespoons Extra-Virgin Olive Oil
- to taste Coarse Ground Salt and Pepper
- 4 sprig Fresh Sage
- Coarse salt (Kosher Salt) to taste
- Coarse Black Pepper to taste
- Small grape tomatoes for garnish* optional

Directions:

1. If you did not buy the Silver Fish (3) gutted and scaled, gut and scale them now. Preheat the oven to 200 degrees C (400 degrees F).
2. Rinse the fish under cold running water and pat dry with paper towel.

Using a sharp knife, cut three diagonal slits into one side of each fish. Season the fish with Coarse Ground Salt and Pepper (to taste), being sure to get into the stomach cavity and the slits. Arrange the fish, slit side up on a lined baking sheet or roasting dish.

3.Wash and chopped Italian Flat-Leaf Parsley (4 sprig), mix with Marjoram Sage and Fresh Basil to make the marinade. Add to a bowl with the Extra-Virgin Olive Oil (2 tablespoons. Zest and juice Lemon (1) and crush the Garlic (6 clove) adding them to the marinade. Season with Coarse Ground Salt and Pepper (to taste) and stir to combine.

4.Place Fish in a baking safe oven dish and sprinkle marinade, salt and pepper to taste on the Silver Fish.

5. Roast the fish at 180 degrees C (350 degrees F) for 20 to 24 minutes until the flesh is no longer translucent and it pulls away easily from the skin.

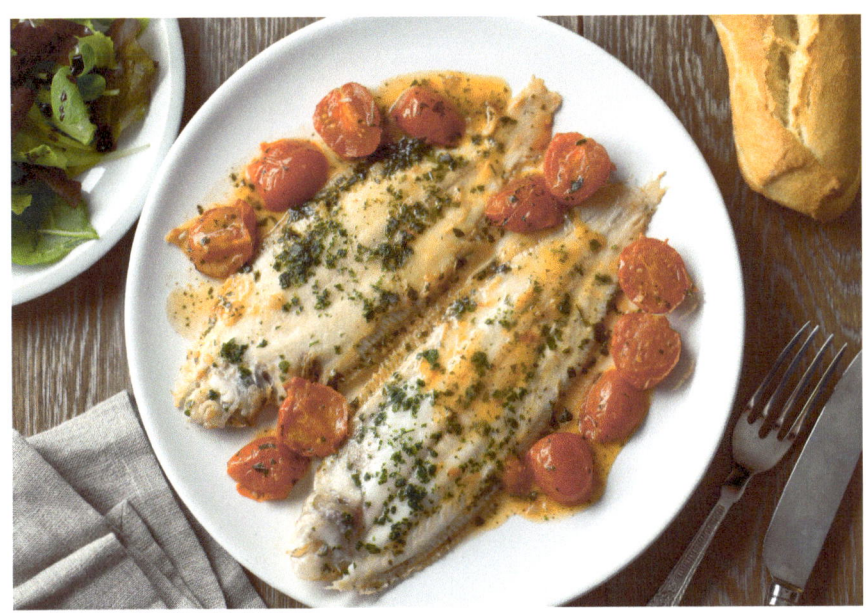

THE SWEET PEPPER CAJUN! TASTY SOULFUL FOOD COOKBOOK!

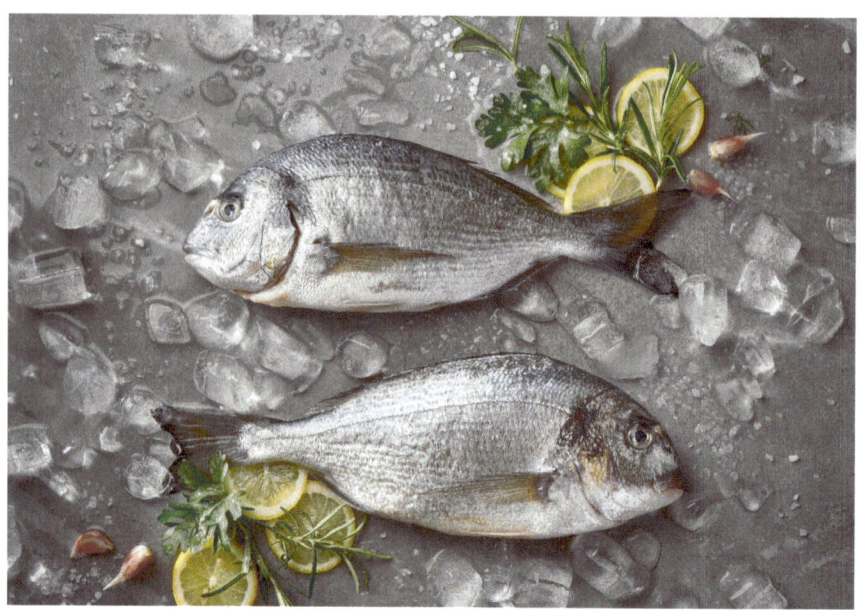

Smoky Collard Greens with Ham!

Ingredients:

- 12 hickory-smoked bacon slices, finely chopped
- 2 medium-size sweet onions, finely chopped
- 3/4 pound smoked ham, chopped
- 6 garlic cloves, finely chopped
- 3 (32-oz.) containers chicken broth
- 3 (1-lb.) packages fresh collard greens, washed and trimmed
- 1/2 teaspoon liquid smoke
- 1 tablespoon sugar
- 1 teaspoon salt
- 3/4 teaspoon pepper

Directions:

Cook bacon in a 10-qt. stockpot over medium heat 10 to 12 minutes or until almost crisp. Add onion, and sauté 8 minutes; add ham and garlic, and sauté 1 minute. Stir in broth and remaining ingredients. Cook 2 hours or to desired degree of tenderness.

　*Optional: Can Use Mixed Greens in this recipe also. Mustard Greens, Kale, Turnip Greens, Chard or Cabbage.

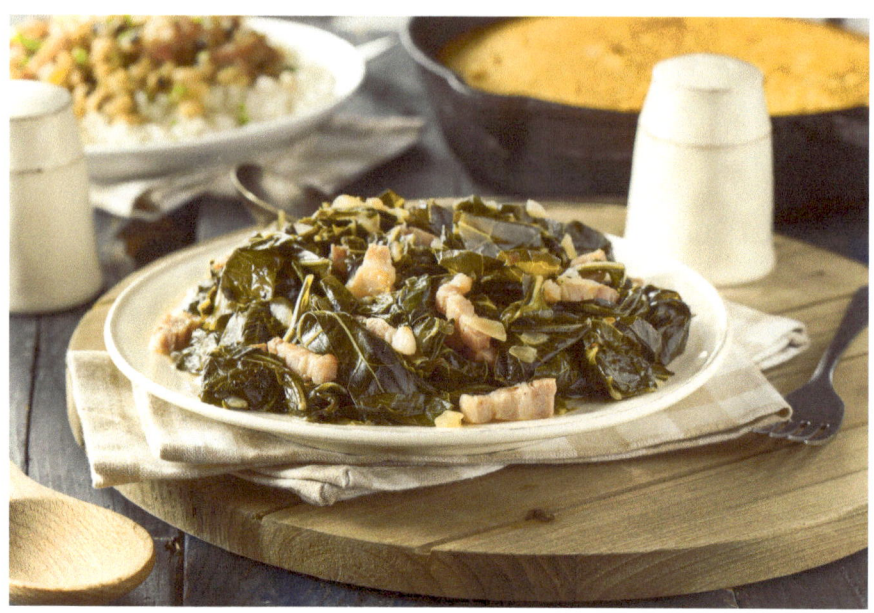

Golden Brown Cornbread!

Ingredients:

- 2 heaping tablespoons butter flavored Crisco
  - 2 eggs
  - 2 cups yellow cornmeal
  - 1 cup all-purpose flour
  - 1 teaspoon sugar
  - whole milk
  - 1/2 teaspoon salt
  - 1/2 teaspoon pepper
  - 1 10" cast iron skillet

Directions:

Mix together cornmeal, flour, sugar, salt and pepper. Add milk until you have the consistency of a cake batter. Add eggs and mix well.
 In the skillet, melt shortening. Move the skillet around until well coated. Pour the remainder into the batter and mix. Pour the batter into the skillet. Bake at 375 for 40 minutes or until light brown.
 *Cornbread will not stick to a seasoned skillet.

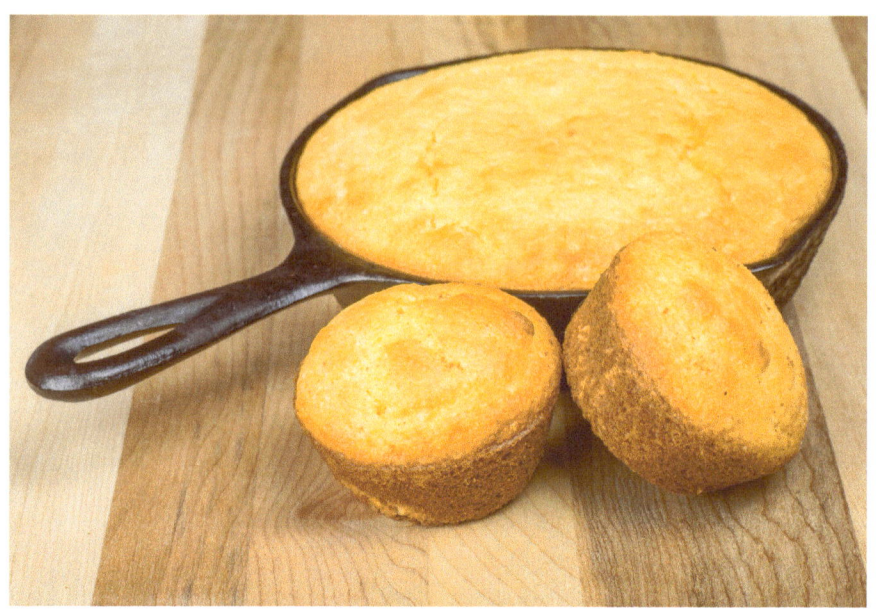

New Year's Good Luck Almond Pound Cake!

Ingredients:

- 1/2 cup slivered almonds
  - 1 cup butter room temperature
  - 1 cup sour cream
  - 4 ounces cream cheese
  - 1 cup butter
  - 2 cups Granulated sugar
  - 6 large eggs
  - 1 teaspoon vanilla extract
  - 1 teaspoon almond extract
  - 3 cups all-purpose flour
  - 1 teaspoon baking powder
  - 1/4 teaspoon salt
  - 1/4 cup powdered sugar *optional topping
  - Optional: whipped cream to serve
  - Optional: Traditionally, the cake is baked with a coin or trinket, and the person who gets that slice is supposed to have good luck for the year ahead. If you are going to insert a coin. Wash coin thoroughly, dry and wrap it in wax paper, once cake batter is made and poured into bundt cake pan, then drop the wax covered coin into the batter.

Directions:

1. Preheat the oven to 325 degrees F and grease a bundt pan well with non-stick spray. Sprinkle slivered almonds in the bottom and on the sides of the bundt pan (you can use the spray to keep the almonds on the sides if you want). Set aside.

2. In a large bowl with an electric or stand mixer, beat butter and cream cheese until smooth and creamy. Gradually add in sugar and sour cream.

3. Add the eggs one at a time and waiting for each one to blend into batter. Add sugar. Beat until all combine add the vanilla extract and almond extract.

4. In a separate bowl blend together flour, baking powder and salt. If you have a flour sifter, sift dry ingredients twice.

5. Once all dry ingredients combine add slowly to the mixer on low speed just until combined. Pour into prepared bundt pan and at this point if you are going to insert a coin. Wash coin thoroughly, dry and wrap it in wax paper then drop the wax paper covered coin into the batter, use a toothpick, Popsicle stick, etc. to push coin well-hidden into the batter. Bake for 50 minutes or until a toothpick inserted near the center comes out clean.

6. Let cool in pan for 10-15 minutes before turning out onto a wire rack to cool to room temperature. *Optional top with powder sugar. Serve with whipped cream and toasted almonds if desired.

NEW YEAR'S GOOD LUCK ALMOND POUND CAKE!

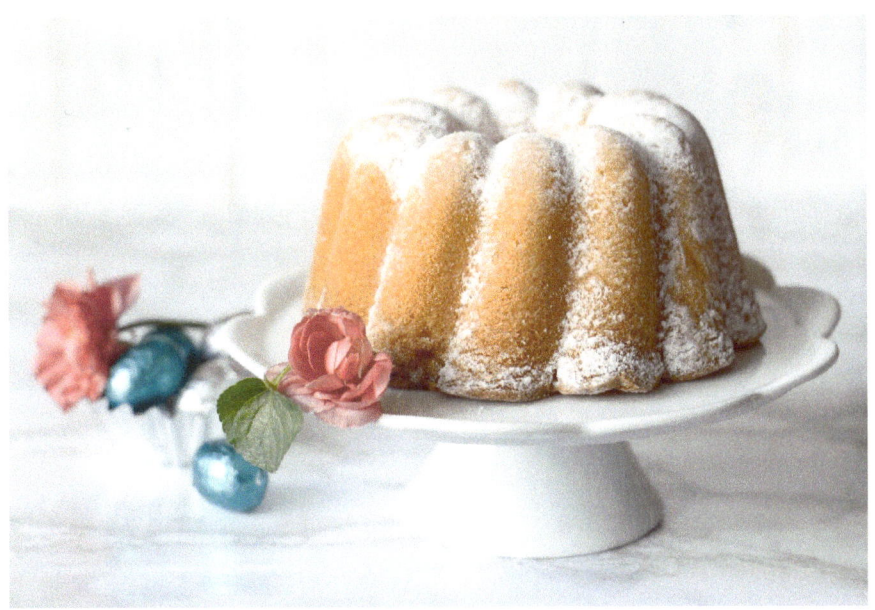

Holiday Appetizer Party!

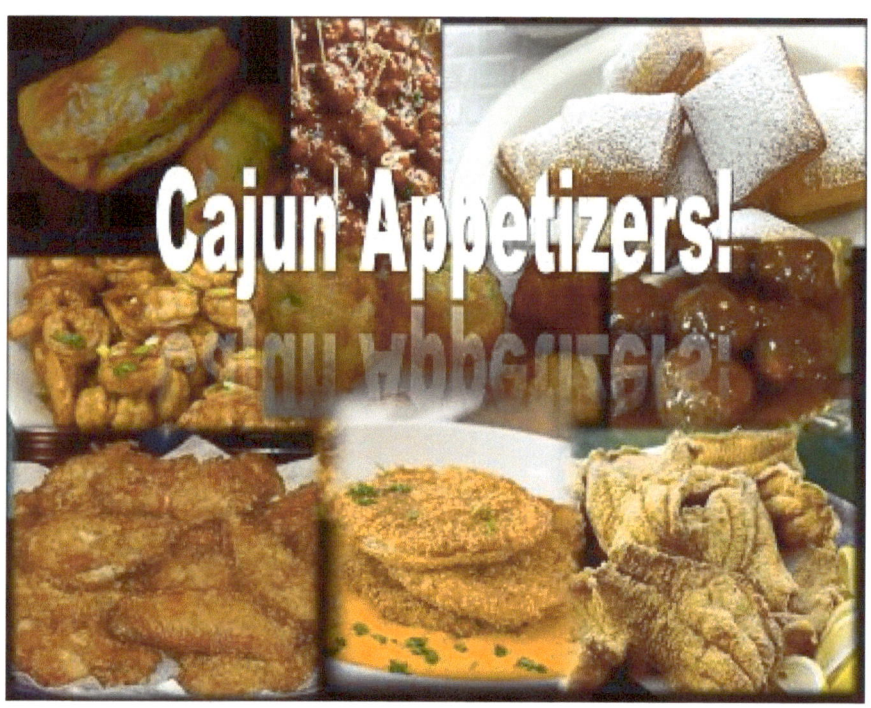

Cajun Mini Crab Cakes!

Ingredients:

8 ounces cream cheese, room temperature
- 3/4 cup finely grated Parmesan cheese, divided
- 1 large egg
- 1/4 cup sour cream
- 1 teaspoon finely grated orange peel
- 1/2 teaspoon finely grated lemon peel
- 4 teaspoons plus 2 tablespoons chopped fresh chives, divided
- 1/4 teaspoon coarse kosher salt
- ¼ teaspoon Slap Ya Mamma seasoning
- Large pinch of cayenne pepper
- 6 ounces fresh lump crab-meat, picked over, patted dry, coarsely shredded
- 1 cup panko (Japanese breadcrumbs)*optional if you want a crunchy outside
- 1/4 cup (1/2 stick) unsalted butter, melted, plus more for pans
- Fresh chives, cut into pieces

Directions:

Using electric mixer, beat cream cheese in medium bowl until smooth. Add 1/4 cup Parmesan and egg; beat to blend. Beat in sour cream, citrus peels, 4 teaspoons chopped chives, coarse Slap Ya Mamma seasoning, salt, and cayenne pepper. Fold in crabmeat.

*Note you can do this ahead. This can be made one day ahead. Cover and chill.

Preheat oven to 350°F. Generously butter 2 mini muffin pans. Toss panko, 1/2 cup Parmesan, and 2 tablespoons chopped chives in small bowl. Drizzle 1/4 cup melted butter over, tossing with fork until evenly moistened. Press 1 rounded tablespoon panko mixture into bottom of each muffin cup, forming crust. Spoon 1 generous tablespoon crab mixture into each cup. Sprinkle rounded teaspoon of panko mixture over each (some may be left over).

Bake crab cakes until golden on top and set, about 30 minutes. Cool in pans 5 minutes. Run knife around each cake and gently lift out of pan. Can be made 2 hours ahead. Arrange on baking sheet; let stand at room temperature. Rewarm in 350°F oven 6 to 8 minutes.

**Arrange on a serving platter and *(optional) sprinkle with chives or parsley.*

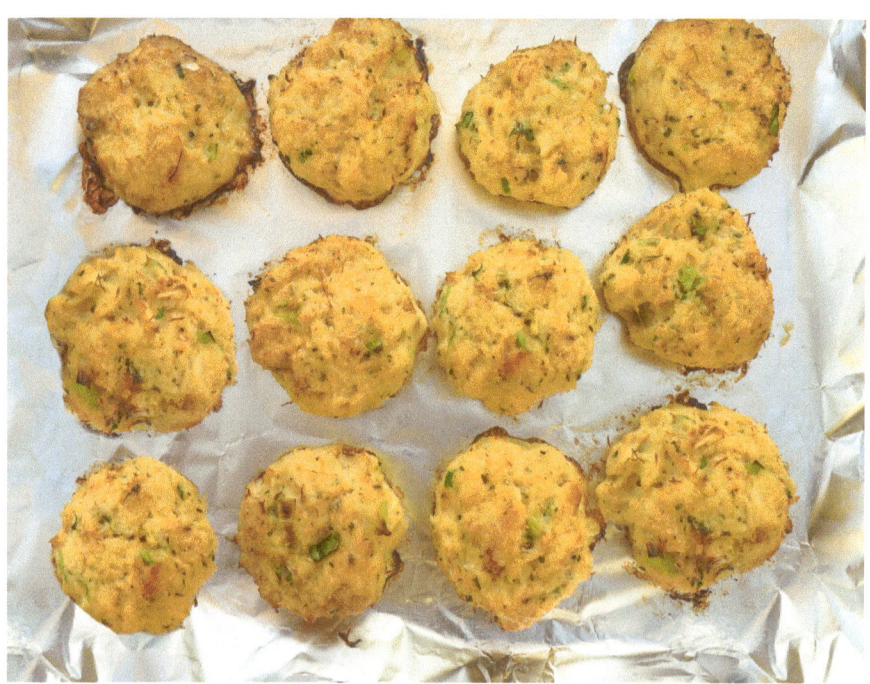

Cajun Stuff Mushrooms!

Ingredients:

Cooking spray, for pan
- 1 1/2 lb. baby mushrooms
- 2 tbsp. butter
- 2 cloves garlic, minced
- 1/4 c. breadcrumbs
- ¼ teaspoon Kosher salt
- ¼ teaspoons Black pepper
- ¼ teaspoon Slap Yo Mamma Cajun Seasoning
- Freshly ground black pepper
- 1/4 c. freshly grated Parmesan, plus more for topping
- 4 oz. cream cheese, softened
- 2 tbsp. freshly chopped parsley
- 1 tbsp. freshly chopped thyme

Directions:

Preheat oven to 400°.

Grease a baking sheet with cooking spray. Remove stems from mushrooms and roughly chop stems. Place mushroom caps on baking sheet.

In a medium skillet over medium heat, melt butter. Add chopped mushrooms stems and cook until most of the moisture is out, 5 minutes. Add garlic and cook until fragrant, 1 minute then add breadcrumbs and let toast slightly, 3 minutes. Season with salt and pepper. Remove from heat and let cool slightly.In a large bowl mix together mushroom stem mixture, Parmesan, cream cheese, parsley, and thyme. Season with salt and pepper.

Fill mushroom caps with filling and sprinkle with more Parmesan.

Bake until mushrooms are soft and the tops are golden, about 20 minutes.

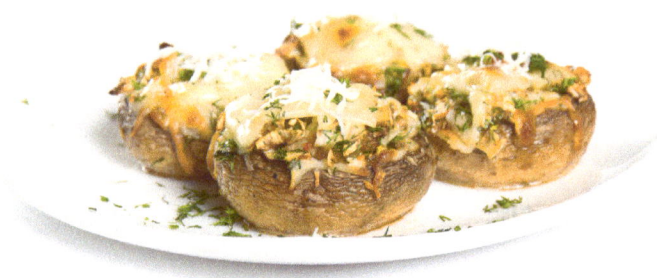

Cajun Oysters Spinach & Cheese!

Ingredients:

- 1/4 cup butter
  - 4 small shallots, finely chopped (about 1/2 cup)
  - 1/3 cup white wine
  - 1 quart loosely-packed baby spinach leaves (about 2 ounces)
  - 1/2 cup cream
  - 1/4 cup grated Parmesan cheese
  - Kosher salt and cracked black pepper
  - 2 teaspoon Slap Yo Mamma Seasoning
  - 24 oysters, shucked
  - 4 tablespoons breadcrumbs

Directions:

Adjust rack to 6 inches below broiler element and preheat broiler to high.

Heat butter in a large nonstick skillet over medium high heat, when butter has melted add shallots and cook, stirring occasionally, until soft, about 4 minutes. Add white wine and baby spinach and cover with a lid. Let steam until spinach has wilted, about 4 minutes, then remove lid and stir until all liquid has evaporated, about 4 minutes longer.

Mix together 1/2 teaspoon Slap Ya Mamma seasoning cracked black pepper and kosher salt. Separate half of season mixture add to breadcrumbs and mix well.

Add cream and Parmesan cheese to the spinach mixture, remove from heat and allow to cool. Sprinkle rest of Seasoning mixture on top.

Divide spinach mixture between shucked oysters (about 1 tablespoon per oyster) then top with breadcrumbs (about 1/2 teaspoon per oyster). Place oysters on roasting pan or sheet pan and place in preheated oven until breadcrumbs are brown, about 6 minutes. Serve immediately.

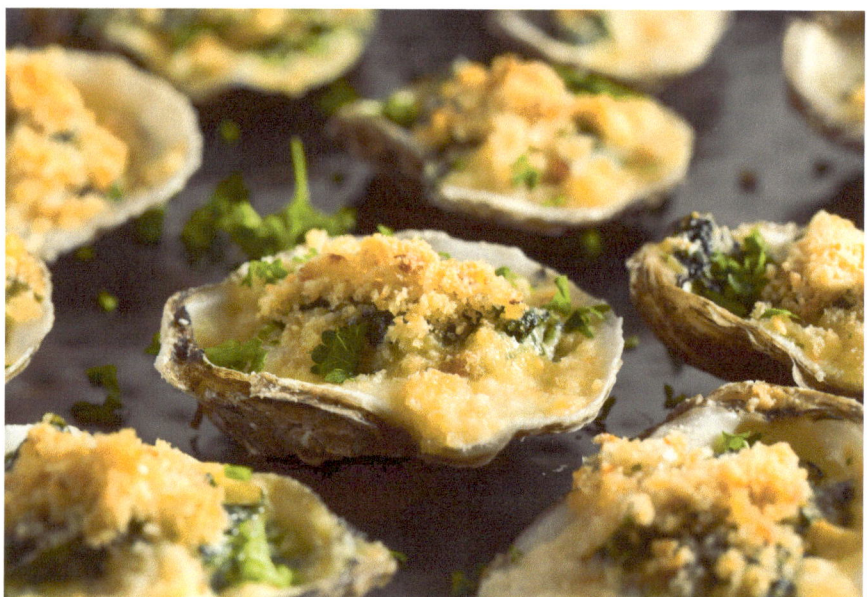

Cajun Ham and Corn Beignets!

Ingredients:

- 1 tablespoon baking powder
  - ½ cup finely diced red onion
  - 1 tablespoon cayenne pepper
  - 10 ounces diced cooked ham
  - ¾ cup milk
  - 4 ears of fresh corn
  - 4 eggs
  - 2 quarts vegetable oil for frying
  - 1 tablespoon Slap Ya Mamma Cajun seasoning
  - 3 cups of all-purpose flour
  - 1 tablespoon baking soda

Directions:

1. In a large heavy pot, preheat the vegetable oil to between 350 degrees F (175 degrees C) and 375 degrees F (190 degrees C).

2. Shuck, wash and dry the corn. Using a sharp knife, shave the ears of corn into a medium sized bowl. Using a cheese grater, scrape any remaining corn and juice into the bowl with the kernels. Discard the scraped cobs.

3. In a mixing bowl, whisk together the eggs and milk. Combine the corn, ham, Slap Yo Mamma seasoning, cayenne pepper, red onion, salt, flour and

baking powder with the egg and milk mixture. Whisk until a firm batter has formed.

4. Slowly drop rounded tablespoonfuls of the batter into the hot oil one at a time. The drops should form a loose layer on the top of the oil. Fry until the drops of batter are dark golden brown. Remove the beignets from the oil and place them on a towel. Check that they are cooked all the way through. If the centers are doughy, lower the heat of the oil and fry the beignets again for 2 or 3 minutes. Repeat this step until all the batter has been used.

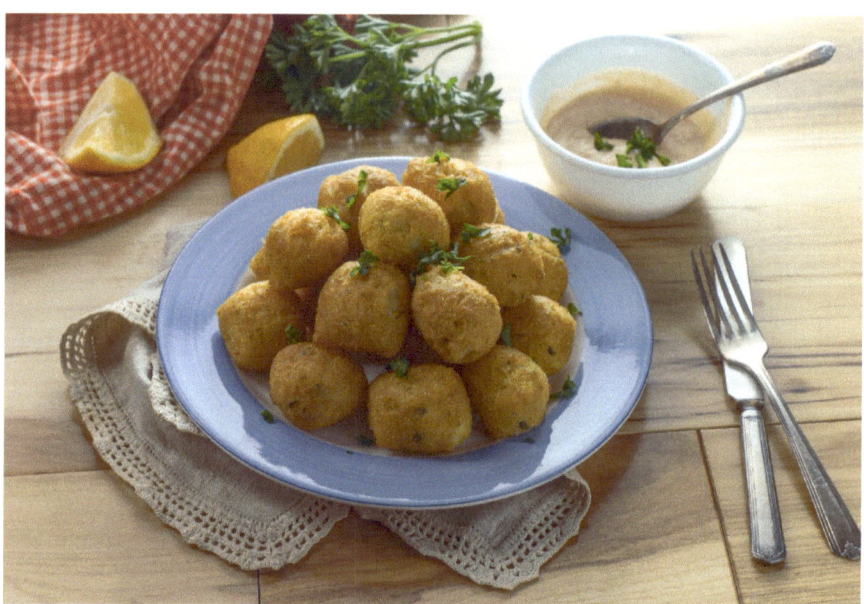

Cajun Crawfish Boulettes!

Cajun Crawfish Boulettes

The word Boulette means little balls in French.

Ingredients:

- 1 (16 ounce) package cooked and peeled whole crawfish tails
  - 1/2 cup chopped onion
  - 1/4 cup chopped green bell pepper
  - 1/4 cup chopped celery
  - 1 1/2 teaspoons minced garlic
  - 5 slices stale white bread, torn into pieces
  - 1 egg
  - 1 teaspoon Slap Ya Mamma Cajun seasoning
  - 1/2 teaspoon black pepper
  - 2 teaspoons Cajun seasoning
  - 2 tablespoons chopped fresh parsley
  - 3 tablespoons thinly sliced green onions
  - 2 quarts vegetable oil for frying
  - 1 1/2 cups dry bread crumbs
  - 1 tablespoon Cajun seasoning

Directions:

1. Place the crawfish tails, chopped onion, bell pepper, celery, garlic, stale bread, and egg into the bowl of a food processor. Add the salt, black pepper, and 2 teaspoons of Cajun seasoning. Cover and pulse until the crayfish mixture is finely chopped. Scrape into a bowl and fold in the parsley and green onions. Cover and refrigerate 1 hour.

2. Heat oil in a deep-fryer or large saucepan to 350 degrees F (175 degrees C). Whisk the bread crumbs and 1 tablespoon of Cajun seasoning together in a bowl; set aside.

3. Form the crawfish mixture into 1 tablespoon-size balls and roll in the bread crumbs. Cook in batches in the hot oil until the balls turn golden brown and begin to float, about 4 minutes. Drain on a paper towel-lined plate and serve hot.

CAJUN CRAWFISH BOULETTES!

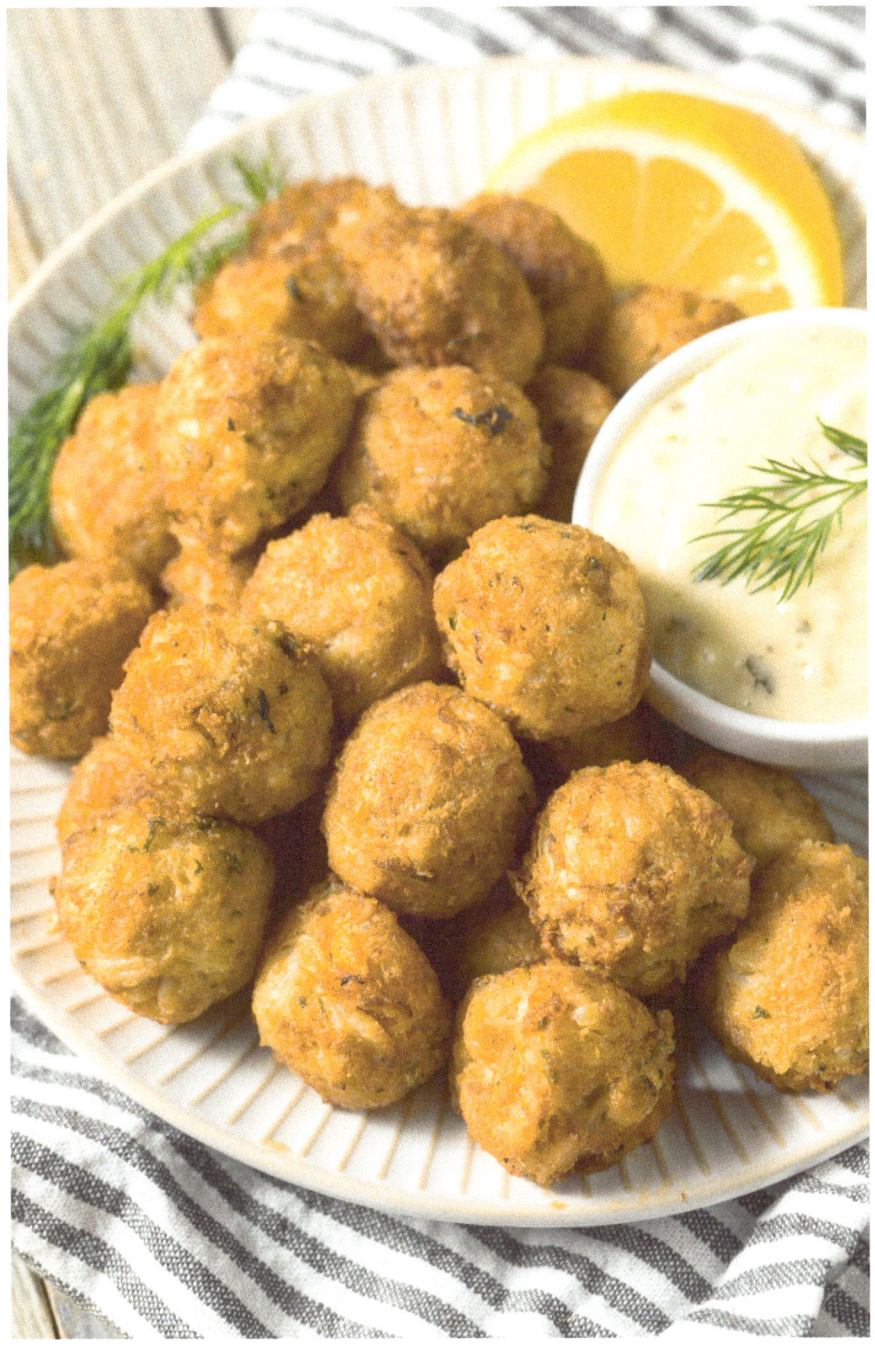

Cajun Spicy Appetizer Meatballs

Ingredients:

These can be made ahead and put in the freezer

- 1 pound lean ground beef
- 1 1/2 teaspoons Louisiana hot sauce *(Frank or Crystal Hot sauce will do fine also)
- 2 tablespoons Slap Ya Mamma Cajun seasoning
- 1 tablespoon Worcestershire sauce
- 1 tablespoon dried parsley
- 1/4 cup finely chopped onion
- 1/4 cup fresh breadcrumbs
- 1/4 cup milk
- 1 egg
- 1/2 cup barbecue sauce
- 1/2 cup peach preserves *(Pineapple or Orange preserve can also be used)

Directions:

1. Preheat oven to 350 degrees F (175 degrees C). Lightly grease a medium baking sheet.
2. In a large bowl, mix thoroughly the ground beef, hot pepper sauce, Slap Ya Mamma Cajun seasoning, Worcestershire sauce, parsley, onion, breadcrumbs, milk, and egg.

3.Form the mixture into golf ball sized meatballs and place on the prepared baking sheet. Bake in preheated oven for 30 to 40 minutes, or until there is no pink left in the middle.

4.In a small bowl, combine the barbecue sauce and peach preserves.

When meatballs are done, place in a serving dish and cover with the barbecue sauce mixture. Toss to coat.

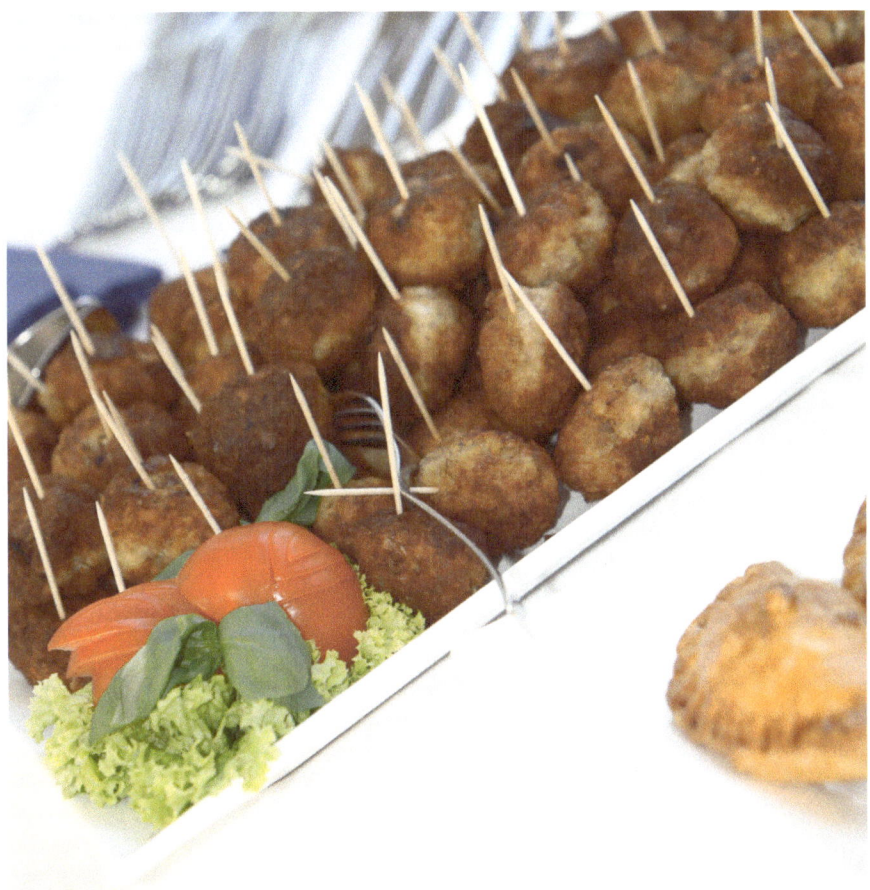

Crispy Oven Friend Cajun Chicken Wings!

Ingredients:
- 4 lbs. of chicken wings or drumsticks
- 2 Tablespoons of baking power
- ¼ cup cornstarch
- 2 teaspoon of Slap Ya Momma Cajun seasoning
- ½ teaspoon black pepper
- ½ teaspoon onion powder
- ½ teaspoon garlic powder
- ¼ teaspoon cayenne pepper
- Non-Stick cooking spray
- ½ cup Louisiana Hot Sauce *(Optional) only if you want wings extra spicy
- Long oven cookie sheet pan

Directions:

Preheat oven to 400 degree

Line a cookie sheet with aluminum foil and spray the foil with non-stick cooking spray. In a large bowl mix together all dry ingredients including the cornstarch. If you are going to make wings extra spicy place ½ cup of Louisiana Hot Sauce in a separate bowl.

1st Dip Spicy wings in hot sauce then dip in dry ingredients mixture, shake off excess and then place wings on top of the foil on the cookie sheet.

Bake for about 25 minutes. Take out the oven and leaving on the hot pan BE CAREFUL and lightly spray the chicken with some of the non-stick spray. Then turn the pieces over and let them go for another 25 minutes. After another 25 minutes check to see if they are done before serving. If not done place chicken back into the over as long as needed to cook through.

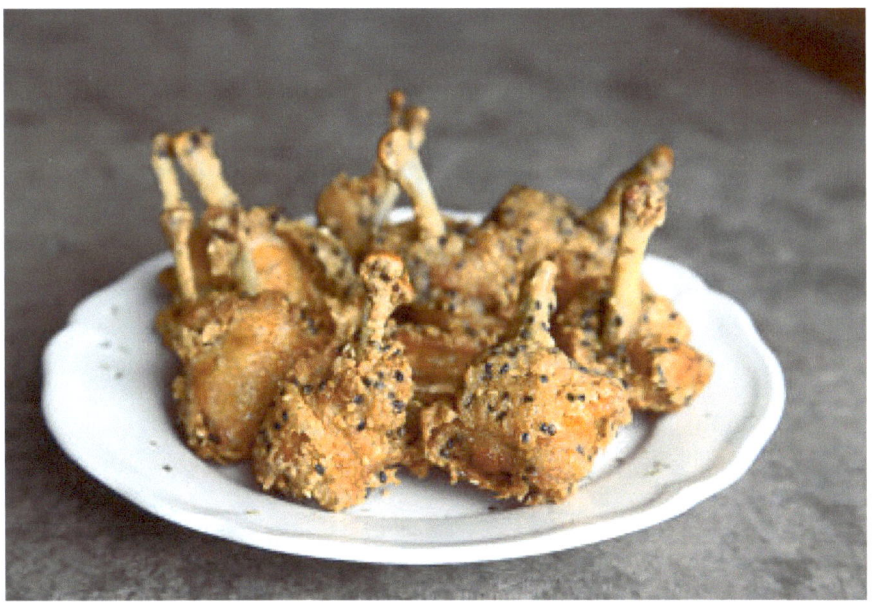

Cajun Pan Roasted Pumpkin Seeds!

Ingredients:

- 1 cup raw pumpkin seed
    - 1/2 teaspoon Slap Ya Mamma Cajun Seasoning
    - 1/4 teaspoon black pepper

Directions:

Heat Skillet over medium heat
- Spray Olive Oil into a skillet
- Pour in 1 cup of raw pumpkin seed, let seed brown on one side. Stir and then add Slap Ya Mamma Cajun seasoning and black pepper.
- Stir continuously until most seeds have toasted a warm brown
- Pour into serving dish and let seeds cool before serving.

CAJUN PAN ROASTED PUMPKIN SEEDS!

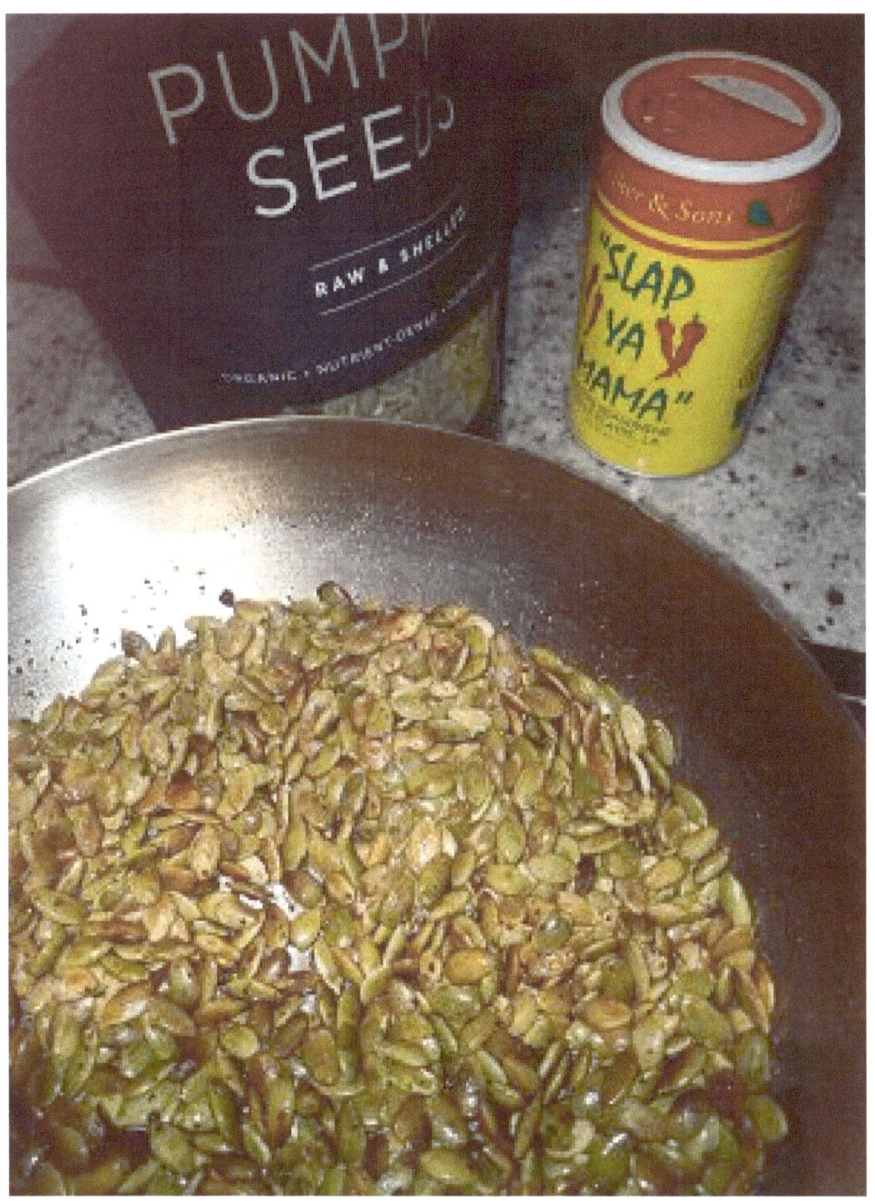

Keep Calm and Cook On!

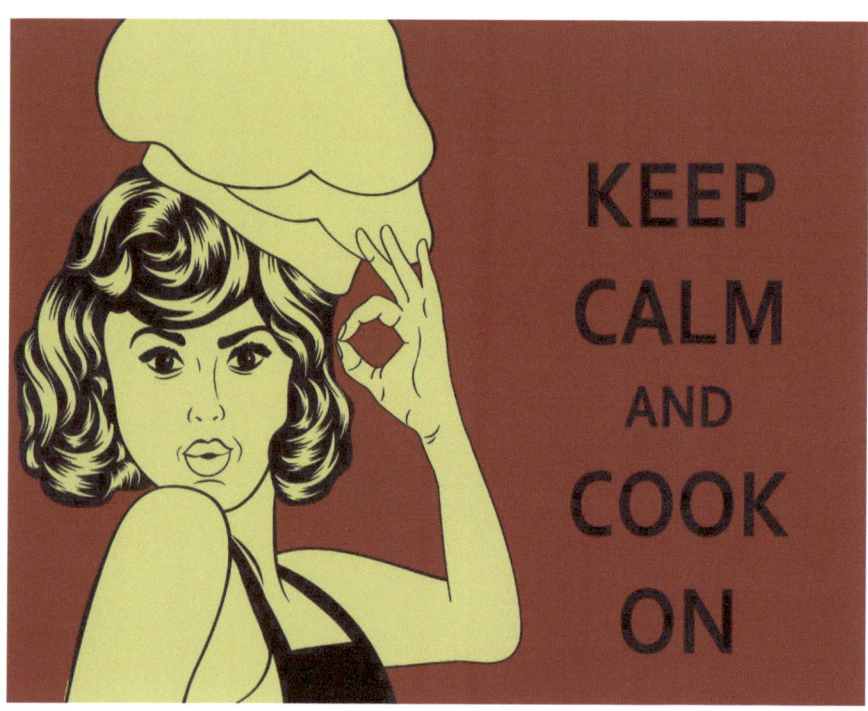

Come Join Us! Taste Our Scrumptious Food!

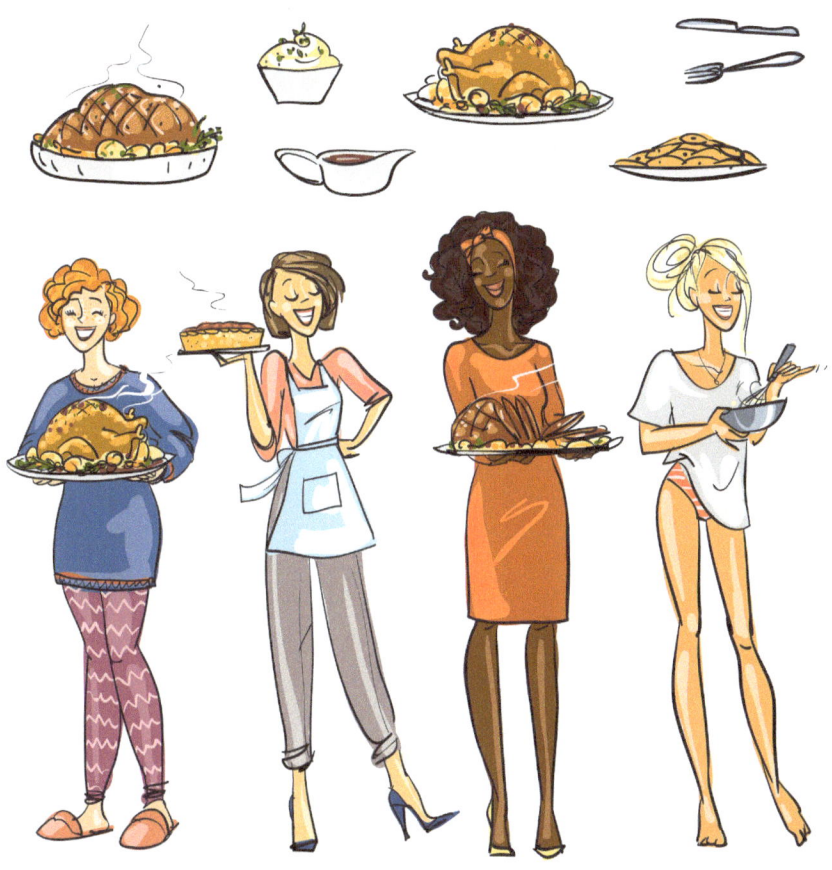

Come join us, grab a seat, fill a bowl, and take a taste of our scrumptious food. We believe food is our common ground and in flavor do we trust! Any Season!

There's an old saying... "Good friends are so very hard to find, and I'm am so grateful that you are mine." This is for you... All of my friends. Thank you.

Young or Old Learning To Cook Can Be Fun!

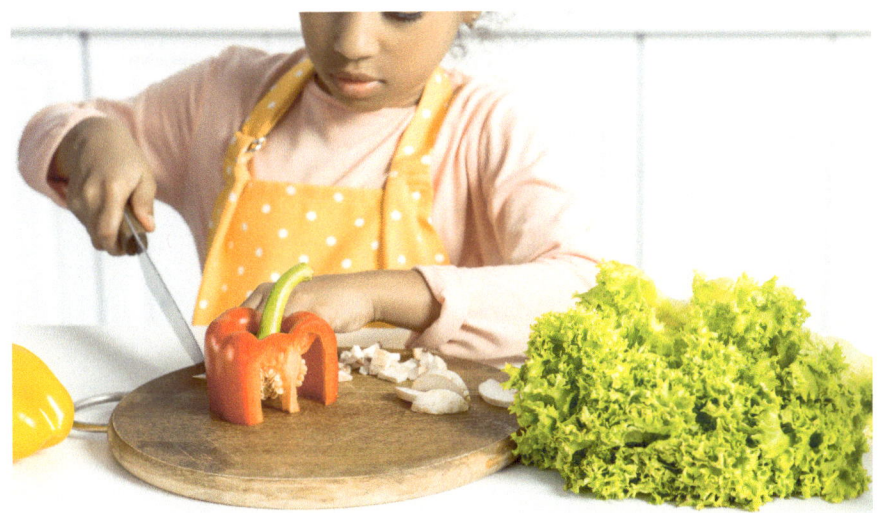

Stay tuned more great recipes to come...

Books by J. A. Jackson

The Deceiver

The Proposition

The Grand Hotel
Lovers, Players, & The Seducer
Lovers, Players, Revenge (Book II)

The Mistress of Desire
& The Orchid Lover Book I
The Mistress of Desire
& The Orchid Lover Book II The Quest!

The Deceiver's Secret

When A Taker Dreams

Diamond at Midnight (Release Winter 2019)

About the Author

J.A. Jackson is the pseudonym for an author, who loves to write deliciously sultry adult romantic, suspenseful, entertaining novels with a unique twist. She lives in an enchanted little house she calls home in the Northern California foothills. Her love for cooking and writing come from her Southern roots of Louisiana and Arkansas.

She spent over ten years working in the non-profit sector where she wrote grants, press releases and contributed many stories to their newsletter. She was their Newsletter editor for over ten years. She loves growing roses, a good pot of hot tea, chocolate, magical stories, suspense stories, ghost stories, and reading Jane Austen again and again in her past time.

Contact: J. A. Jackson P. O. Box 1494, Clovis CA 93613

Email: jerreecejackson@yahoo.com

You can connect with me on:
- http://jerreeceannjackson.blogspot.com
- https://twitter.com/jerreece
- https://www.facebook.com/JerreeceJackson/?ref=bookmarks
- https://www.amazon.com/-/e/B01ISNR0B2

Subscribe to my newsletter:
- https://mailchi.mp/ddf9555be2a4/theauthorjajackson

Also by J. A. Jackson

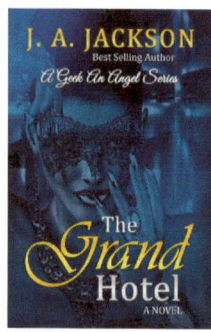

The Grand Hotel

Louis La Cour thought he knew everything there was to know about a scheming, want to be beauty queen's mother.

But knowing the difference between a diabolical mastermind and a monster hell-bent on destroying the lives of everyone around them is a whole other matter. Love, lust, and hatred are basic elements of the story when shattered dreams turn trust and loyalty into desperation, deception, and dishonor.